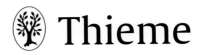

Endoscopy of the Upper GI Tract

A Training Manual

Berthold Block, M.D.
Braunschweig
Germany

Guido Schachschal, M.D.
Universitäts-Klinikum Charité
Berlin
Germany

Hartmut Schmidt, M.D.
Universitäts-Klinikum Charité
Berlin
Germany

774 illustrations
56 tables

Thieme
Stuttgart · New York

Library of Congress Cataloging-in-Publication Data is available from the publisher

This book is an authorized translation of the German edition published and copyrighted 2003 by Georg Thieme Verlag, Stuttgart, Germany. Title of the German edition: Der Gastroskopie-Trainer: Schritt-für-Schritt-Anleitungen für die Ösophago-, Gastro- und Duodenoskopie

Translator: Terry C Telger, Fort Worth, TX, USA

© 2004 Georg Thieme Verlag,
Rüdigerstrasse 14, 70469 Stuttgart, Germany
http://www.thieme.de
Thieme New York, 333 Seventh Avenue,
New York, NY 10001 USA
http://www.thieme.com

Typesetting by primustype Hurler, Notzingen
Printed in Germany by Grammlich, Pliezhausen

ISBN 3-13-136731-8 (GTV)
ISBN 1-58890-239-0 (TNY)   1 2 3 4 5

Preface

Attempts to look into human body orifices and body cavities date back to antiquity. Most of these efforts met with little success because of poor illumination. A breakthrough came in 1806 when Philip Bozzini introduced his *Lichtleiter* ("light conductor"), which supplied at least a theoretical solution to the problem. Bozzini was the first to envision the future application of endoscopes in urology, gynecology, and gastroenterology and the eventual development of laparoscopy.

Adolf Kussmaul introduced the rigid gastroscope in the 1890s. The gastroscopes used during the first half of the 20th century were semirigid devices in which lens systems transmitted the image to an eyepiece. A major advance came in the mid-20th century, when Basil Hirschowitz developed a flexible fiberoptic endoscope. But even this technology appears to have been superseded by the development of video endoscopy and, more recently, by wireless capsule endoscopy.

As endoscopy has evolved, the instruments have become more flexible and their outer diameters smaller, making the examination much easier for both the endoscopist and the patient. Today, upper gastrointestinal endoscopy is the most rewarding procedure for investigating complaints of the upper gastrointestinal tract. Visual inspection, specimen collection, and any necessary interventions can be carried out in the same sitting. Upper gastrointestinal endoscopy is safe and easy to perform for experienced endoscopists.

The quality of the examination depends upon the interplay between the endoscopic technique and the interpretation of the images. Anyone who is learning endoscopy is bound to encounter technical difficulties at first. For this reason, we have provided ample didactic information to supplement the atlas portions of this book.

Endoscopic interventional procedures have been practiced for more than 30 years. The range of endoscopic treatment options is constantly expanding, and examiners are often expected to perform these interventions in the early phase of their endoscopic training. Established therapeutic procedures are described in some detail, therefore.

We hope to provide our readers with an easy-to-use, comprehensive introduction to the method and its capabilities, and we wish them much success and satisfaction in the practice of gastrointestinal endoscopy.

Braunschweig and Berlin, spring 2004

Berthold Block
Guido Schachschal
Hartmut Schmidt

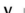

Acknowledgments

We wish to recognize all those who contributed to the success of this book. We thank the following colleagues for providing endoscopic images:

Dr. med. Dirk Bandorski, Fulda Medical Center, Medical Clinic II, Pacelliallee 4, 36043 Fulda.

Dr. med. Christian Bömecke, Agnes Karl Hospital, Hildesheimer Strasse 158, 30880 Hanover–Laatzen.

Dr. med. Thomas Koch, Medical Clinic I, St. Walburga Hospital, Schederweg 12, 59872 Meschede. (*http://www.info-endoskopie.de*)

Dr. med. Werner Schmidtbaur, Augsburg Medical Center, Medical Clinic III, Stenglinstrasse 2, 68156 Augsburg.

We are grateful to Mr. Horst Wesche, of the German Photographic Society in Hanover, for kindly providing the images pertaining to duodenal tube placement.

We thank Mrs. Stephanie Gay and Mr. Bert Sender of Bremen for turning our rough drawings into superb illustrations. Some of the graphics were based on drawings by Mr. Michael Gradias of Wolfenbüttel (originally done for the *Teaching Atlas of Gastroscopy*. Stuttgart: Thieme; 1997).

We thank the excellent staff at our endoscopy unit at the Charité Hospital for their help and patience in obtaining the endoscopic images: Mrs. Ingrid Olerich, Mrs. Silvia Meinert, Mrs. Dagmar Nitschke, Mrs. Martina Linser, Mrs. Marion Doss, Mrs. Marion Strelow, Mrs. Grit Gartmann, Mrs. Annette Klameth, and Mr. Frank Maltzahn.

It is one thing to write text and obtain endoscopic images, but it is quite another to turn them into a book. We are grateful to the staff at Thieme Medical Publishers for presenting our text and endoscopic images in such an exquisite form. We thank Dr. Antje Schönplug and Mrs. Marion Holzer for their tireless efforts. We also thank Dr. Markus Becker, who contributed so much to the success of this book during all phases of its planning and production.

Berthold Block
Guido Schachschal
Hartmut Schmidt

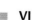

Abbreviations

ALA	aminolevulinic acid		LES	lower esophageal sphincter
AP	anteroposterior		MALT	mucosa-associated lymphoid tissue
ARDS	adult respiratory distress syndrome		NPO	nothing by mouth
CMV	cytomegalovirus		NSAIDs	nonsteroidal anti-inflammatory drugs
CT	computed tomography		PCR	polymerase chain reaction
ECG	echocardiogram		PEG	percutaneous endoscopic gastrostomy
EGD	esophagogastroduodenoscopy		PEJ	percutaneous endoscopic jejunostomy
ENT	ear, nose, and throat		PPI	proton pump inhibitors
GAVE	gastric antral venous ectasia		TIPS	transjugular intrahepatic portosystemic shunting
GI	gastrointestinal (only in "upper GI endoscopy")		TTC	through-the-channel
HSV	herpes simplex virus		TTS	through-the-scope

Contents

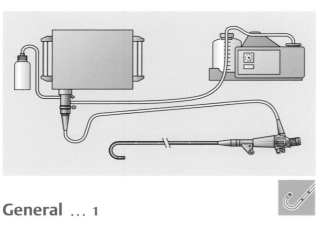

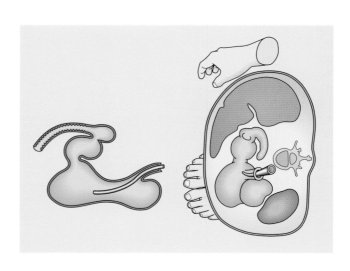

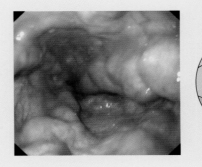
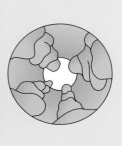

3.1 Pathological Findings: Esophagus ... 58

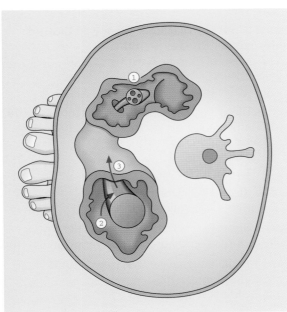

Contents

3.2 Pathological Findings: Stomach ... 94

3.3 Pathological Findings: Duodenum ... 130

4 Interventional Procedures and Extended Endoscopic Examination Methods ... 142

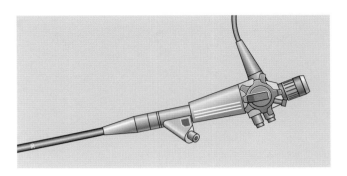

Contents

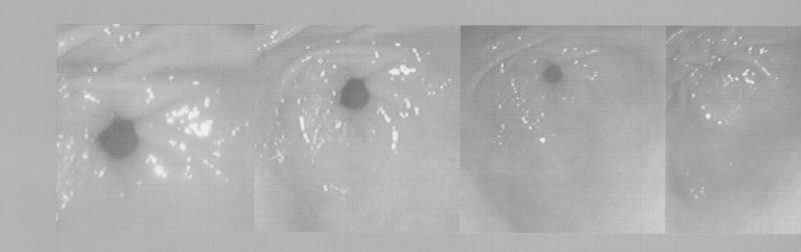

1 General

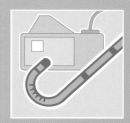

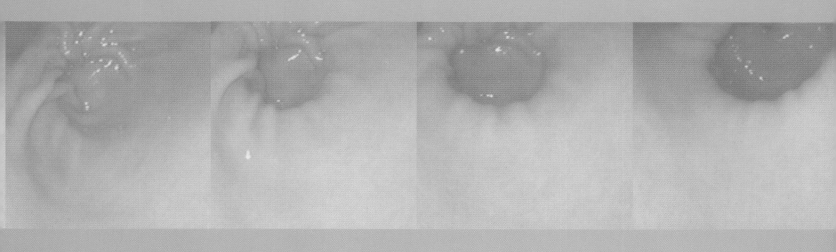

Indications and Contraindications

Upper gastrointestinal endoscopy, known also as upper GI endoscopy or esophagogastroduodenoscopy (EGD), is the method of choice for examining the esophagus, stomach, and duodenum. In one sitting, it permits the gross visual inspection of the upper gastrointestinal tract, the collection of tissue and fluid samples, as well as elective and emergency therapeutic interventions. It can be performed quickly and safely with good patient tolerance and without extensive patient preparations. The requirements in terms of equipment and operator proficiency are relatively modest.

■ Indications

Upper GI endoscopy has a broad range of indications. It is used to confirm or exclude a particular diagnosis in patients with upper gastrointestinal complaints, to monitor the progression of a known disease, and for staging in patients with a systemic disease (Fig. 1.**1**).

■ Contraindications

An absolute contraindication to elective upper GI endoscopy is lack of informed consent from a mentally competent patient. Relative contraindications are organ perforations and states of cardiac or respiratory decompensation (Fig. 1.**2**).

Fig. 1.1 Indications

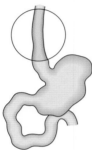

a Dysphagia, swallowing difficulties, retrosternal pain

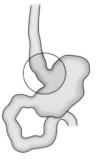

b Upper abdominal pain, heartburn, Barrett esophagus, peptic stricture, achalasia

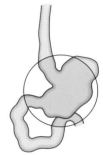

c Nausea, vomiting, anorexia, fullness, hematemesis, weight loss, pernicious anemia, diarrhea (sprue)

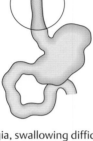

d Unexplained aspiration, chronic cough

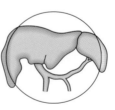

e Portal hypertension

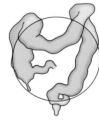

f Chronic inflammatory bowel disease, familial polyposis syndromes

---

Fig. 1.2 Relative contraindications

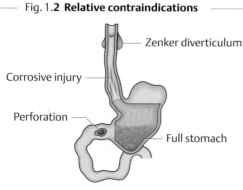

Zenker diverticulum

Corrosive injury

Perforation

Full stomach

a Zenker diverticula, corrosive ingestion, perforation, full stomach

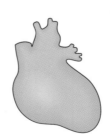

b Heart failure, acute myocardial ischemia

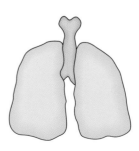

c Respiratory failure

General

Risks and Complications: Cardiac and Pulmonary

The rate of serious complications in upper GI endoscopy is small and is measured in tenths of a percent (Table 1.1). Reports based on larger reviews show that the mortality rate is less than 0.01 %.

It should be emphasized that most complications do not involve the gastrointestinal tract itself but consist of respiratory or cardiovascular incidents, especially in sick or sedated patients (Table 1.2).

Complications can result from local anesthesia, sedation, or the endoscopy itself. They consist mainly of respiratory and cardiovascular events, mechanical injuries, hemorrhages, and infections.

Table 1.1 **Complication rates in upper GI endoscopy**

Complication	Complication rate	Percentage of all complications
Cardiac	1:2000	60 %
Pulmonary	1:4000	30 %
Perforation, bleeding	1:15 000	9 %
Infection	1:50 000	1 %

Table 1.2 **Risk factors and high-risk patients**

► Advanced age
► NYHA class III–IV heart failure
► Grade III–IV aortic stenosis
► Severe pulmonary disease
► Bleeding tendency
  (Quick prothrombin < 50 %, thrombopenia < 50 000/µL)
► Anemia (Hb < 8 g/dL)
► Emergency procedures

■ Local Anesthesia

Anesthetic throat sprays have the potential to incite an allergic reaction, produce cardiac side effects, and promote aspiration. The overall risk of complications from pharyngeal anesthesia is approximately 1:10 000. The risk of fatal complications is considerably lower.

■ Sedation and Analgesia

Benzodiazepines. The use of benzodiazepines is often associated with a decrease in arterial oxygen saturation, but this is rarely significant. The risk is increased in older patients, patients with chronic respiratory failure, coronary heart disease, or hepatic insufficiency, and in emergency endoscopy.

The principal risks are a fall in blood pressure and hypoxemia-induced cardiac arrhythmia. Myocardial infarctions during endoscopy are rare. Respiratory complications can range from hypoventilation to apnea. The most common problem is aspiration. Sedation is believed to be the principal risk factor for aspiration pneumonia.

Narcotics. The use of narcotic analgesics, such as Pethidine, can lead to hypotension and bradycardia.

■ Cardiac Complications

Approximately 50 % of the complications that occur in upper GI endoscopy are cardiac in nature. They consist of heart rate changes, arrhythmias, and repolarization abnormalities. The mortality rate of cardiac complications ranges from 1:20 000 to 1:50 000.

Arrhythmias. The most common arrhythmias are tachycardia and extrasystoles, which usually have no clinical significance and are spontaneously reversible. Bradycardia is observed in fewer than 5 % of patients. Significant tachyarrhythmias are also rare.

Repolarization abnormalities. These occur predominantly in patients with coronary heart disease. They reflect a myocardial ischemia, usually clinically silent, that is caused by arterial hypoxia due to the increased cardiac work load.

■ Respiratory Complications

Respiratory complications consist of hypoventilation, apnea, and aspiration, usually in connection with premedication. Their overall incidence is low, however. The mortality rate is less than 1:50 000.

Risks and Complications: Gastrointestinal

■ Perforation and Bleeding

Although perforation and bleeding from gastroscopy are the complications that patients fear the most, they account for less than 10% of all complications in diagnostic endoscopy.

The most common sites of perforation, in descending order of frequency, are the esophagus, hypopharynx, duodenum, and stomach. Predisposing factors are diverticula, severe cervical spondylosis, and endoscopic interventions such as dilation, prosthesis insertion, and laser therapy (Fig. 1.3). Severe postbiopsy bleeding during or after endoscopy is rare.

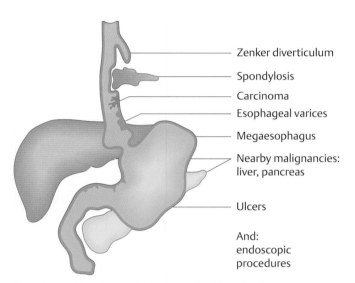

Zenker diverticulum

Spondylosis

Carcinoma

Esophageal varices

Megaesophagus

Nearby malignancies: liver, pancreas

Ulcers

And: endoscopic procedures

Fig. 1.3 **Perforation and bleeding.** Predisposing factors

■ Infection

The risk of clinically overt infection after upper GI endoscopy is extremely small, but does exist. Bacteremia is a common occurrence, however. Three factors are relevant in the pathogenesis of infection: the transmission of infectious organisms, the nature of the procedure, and patient-associated risks (Table 1.3).

Disease Transmission

The direct transmission of microorganisms from patient to patient by contaminated endoscopes has been described for *Salmonellae*, mycobacteria, *Helicobacter pylori*, hepatitis B virus, and other pathogens. The endoscopic transmission of HIV infection has not yet been definitely confirmed.

Bacteremia is not uncommon after endoscopy (up to 5% of cases) but usually has no clinical significance. The endoscope itself can be a reservoir for pathogenic microorganisms (including pseudomonas). Potential sources of infection are contaminated water bottles and the endoscope channels that are more difficult to access and clean. Meticulous cleaning and disinfection after each endoscopy and before the first endoscopy of the day are essential elements of risk management.

Nature of the Procedure

It is clear that procedures that inflict mucosal injuries are associated with a higher infection risk than a simple, uncomplicated endoscopy. Antibiotic prophylaxis should be used liberally in cases deemed to be at risk.

Patient-Associated Risks

These risks consist mainly of cardiac anomalies, prosthetic valves, and immunosuppression. The regimen shown in Table 1.4 is recommended for general antibiotic prophylaxis but should be tailored to suit individual clinical requirements.

Table 1.3 **Endoscopically induced infection: risk factors**

Transmission of infectious organisms
▶ From the previously examined patient
▶ Endogenous transmission (bacteremia)
▶ Contaminated endoscope

Nature of the procedure
▶ Simple endoscopy
▶ Tissue or fluid sampling
▶ Polypectomy
▶ Injection
▶ Bougie or balloon dilation, stenting, prosthesis insertion

Patient
▶ Cardiac valve defects
▶ Artificial heart valve
▶ Indwelling venous catheter, port
▶ Immunosuppression
▶ Hematological disease
▶ Immune-suppressing drugs
▶ HIV infection
▶ Advanced liver or kidney disease

Table 1.4 **Antibiotic prophylaxis in high-risk patients**

Diagnostic endoscopy
▶ Ampicillin, 2 g orally 30–60 min before the procedure
▶ Ampicillin, 1.5 g orally 6 hours after the procedure

Interventional endoscopy
▶ Add before the procedure: 80 mg gentamycin i. v. or 2 g cefotaxime i. v.

In patients allergic to penicillin
▶ Clindamycin, 600 mg orally 1 hour before the procedure

General

Endoscopy Suite: Facilities and Staff

The size, equipment, and organization of the endoscopy suite are determined by the frequency of endoscopic procedures and the requirements that they must satisfy.

■ Procedure Room

Room. The procedure room should be large enough to accommodate all necessary instruments and equipment, the recumbent patient, and at least two other people. The room should have bright lighting that can be dimmed when necessary. Access to fresh air is desirable. Cleaning requirements should be considered during planning and setup of the room. A toilet and recovery area should be easily accessible.

Equipment. The minimum equipment and instruments needed for an endoscopy suite are the endoscope and supply unit, a cleaning area, examination table, sinks, emergency equipment, storage space for drugs, disposables, and accessories, and places for the patient and examiner to sit down.

■ Staff

Assistants. Although an experienced endoscopist can work successfully with inexperienced assistants, specially trained assistants are essential for more complex examinations and for procedures in high-risk patients. An experienced, efficient endoscopy nurse is an invaluable asset to the beginner.

Functions. The functions of the endoscopy nursing staff include setting up the necessary equipment, preparing the patient, assisting the endoscopist in inserting and advancing the instrument, observing the patient, comforting and reassuring the patient during the procedure, assisting with specimen collection, monitoring the patient's recovery, and cleaning and processing the equipment. The nursing staff should know the basic rules of emergency care in the event that complications arise. Endoscopy team members with a negative hepatitis A or B immune status should be immunized without delay.

■ Endoscopy Unit

The endoscopy unit in the strict sense consists of the supply unit, the endoscope, and the cleaning area (Fig. 1.4).

Supply Unit

The supply unit consists of a light source, a compressed air pump for delivering air and water, a suction pump, and a video processor (for video endoscopy). These units converge at the supply plug of the endoscope.

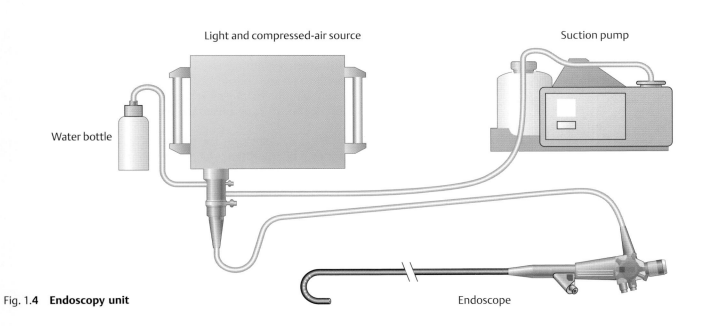

Light and compressed-air source

Suction pump

Water bottle

Fig. 1.4 **Endoscopy unit**

Endoscope

Endoscopy Suite: Endoscope

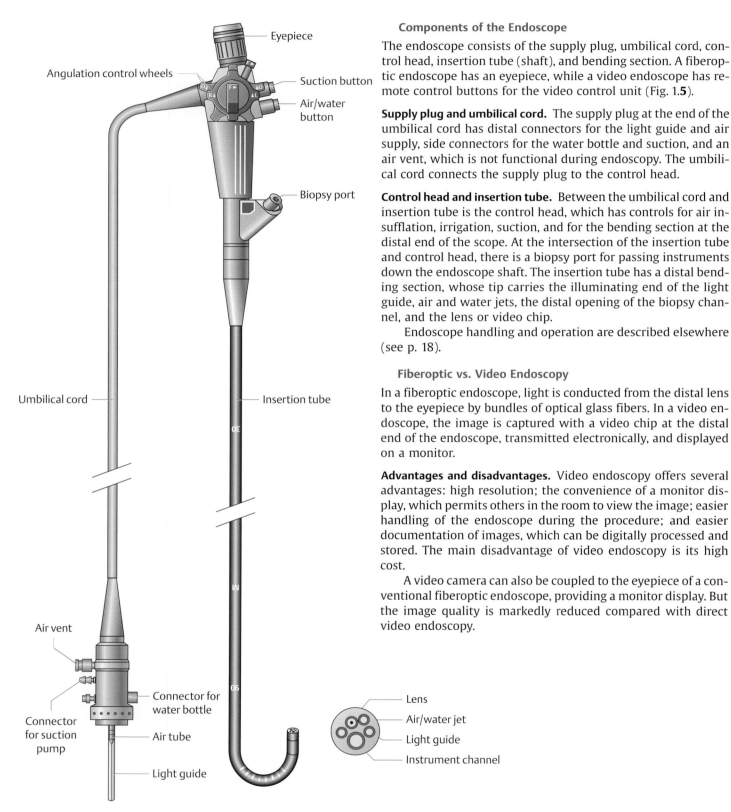

Fig. 1.5 **Endoscope**

Components of the Endoscope

The endoscope consists of the supply plug, umbilical cord, control head, insertion tube (shaft), and bending section. A fiberoptic endoscope has an eyepiece, while a video endoscope has remote control buttons for the video control unit (Fig. 1.5).

Supply plug and umbilical cord. The supply plug at the end of the umbilical cord has distal connectors for the light guide and air supply, side connectors for the water bottle and suction, and an air vent, which is not functional during endoscopy. The umbilical cord connects the supply plug to the control head.

Control head and insertion tube. Between the umbilical cord and insertion tube is the control head, which has controls for air insufflation, irrigation, suction, and for the bending section at the distal end of the scope. At the intersection of the insertion tube and control head, there is a biopsy port for passing instruments down the endoscope shaft. The insertion tube has a distal bending section, whose tip carries the illuminating end of the light guide, air and water jets, the distal opening of the biopsy channel, and the lens or video chip.

Endoscope handling and operation are described elsewhere (see p. 18).

Fiberoptic vs. Video Endoscopy

In a fiberoptic endoscope, light is conducted from the distal lens to the eyepiece by bundles of optical glass fibers. In a video endoscope, the image is captured with a video chip at the distal end of the endoscope, transmitted electronically, and displayed on a monitor.

Advantages and disadvantages. Video endoscopy offers several advantages: high resolution; the convenience of a monitor display, which permits others in the room to view the image; easier handling of the endoscope during the procedure; and easier documentation of images, which can be digitally processed and stored. The main disadvantage of video endoscopy is its high cost.

A video camera can also be coupled to the eyepiece of a conventional fiberoptic endoscope, providing a monitor display. But the image quality is markedly reduced compared with direct video endoscopy.

Endoscopy Suite: Accessories

■ Endoscopic Accessories

The great advantage of endoscopy lies in the option of using both diagnostic and therapeutic instruments in one session. The necessary endoscopic accessories will depend on the requirements of the endoscopy department. Standard accessories consist of irrigation and suction tubes, cytology brushes, biopsy forceps, foreign-body retrieval forceps, and injection needles. Optional accessories include polypectomy snares, extraction baskets, dilators, and dilation sets.

■ Emergency Equipment

Upper GI endoscopy should be performed only if proper emergency supplies are within reach. The items listed in Table 1.5 should be available.

Necessary emergency medications are listed in Table 1.6.

■ Documentation of Findings

The cornerstone of documentation is the written endoscopy report. Images documenting abnormal findings and even normal findings in selected cases are a desirable adjunct to the written report.

Image documentation. Selected images can be printed out on a video printer. Documentation on videotape can provide a complete record of the examination procedure and findings, but videotapes can be costly to archive. A standard written report that gives a brief description of all inspected areas, including normal findings, is unsurpassed for its reproducibility and its value as a baseline for future examinations.

Guidelines for endoscopic reporting are provided on page 182 ff.

Table 1.**5**   **Emergency equipment**

▶ Suction apparatus
▶ Oxygen
▶ Intubation set
▶ Ventilation bag
▶ Defibrillator
▶ Pulse oximeter
▶ ECG monitor
▶ Sphygmomanometer
▶ Indwelling venous cannula
▶ Sengstaken tube
▶ Sclerosant

Table 1.**6**   **Emergency medications (selection)**

Atropine	Atropine, 0.5-mg ampules
Epinephrine	Suprarenin, 1-mL ampules 1:1000
Flumazenil	Anexate, 0.5-mg ampules
Lidocaine	Xylocaine, 0.5% 5 mL
Naloxone	Narcanti, 0.4-mg ampules
Theophylline	Euphyllin, 240-mg ampules
Prednisolone	Solu-Decortin, 250-mg ampules
Nitro spray	Nitrolingual Spray
Nifedipine	Adalat capsules
Clemastine	Tavegil, 2-mg ampules
Infusion solutions	

Preparations for Endoscopy: Informed Consent

■ Disclosure and Informed Consent

Disclosure should be taken very seriously. It is generally known that the great majority of lawsuits brought by patients against physicians stem from inadequate disclosure rather than treatment errors. Despite its relatively high tolerance and low complication risks, upper GI endoscopy is still an invasive examination. The patient should sign a consent form confirming that the physician has fully explained the nature and risks of the procedure, and the consent form should accurately reflect the information that the patient has received.

General Policies

- ▶ Disclosure is provided by a physician.
- ▶ Disclosure should be given at least 24 hours prior to the examination.
- ▶ Disclosure is given verbally and in writing (aided by a standard information sheet).
- ▶ The consent form should reflect the information that has been disclosed.
- ▶ The patient willingly consents to the procedure in writing.

Exceptions

- ▶ Disclosure may be waived for patients who are not verbally responsive.
- ▶ Disclosure may be waived in emergencies and for incompetent patients.

Content of Disclosure

Adequate disclosure should include the reasons for performing the examination and the details of the procedure itself, patient-associated risks and special circumstances, the risks of the examination and of medications used during the procedure, and patient instructions before and after the examination.

General information about the procedure

- ▶ Reason for the examination
- ▶ Nature and conduct of the examination
- ▶ Alternatives
- ▶ Possible consequences of refusing the procedure
- ▶ Risks and discomfort

Patient

- ▶ Patient risk factors
- ▶ Allergies
- ▶ Prior illnesses
- ▶ Bleeding tendency
- ▶ Dental status
- ▶ Prior surgery
- ▶ Medications that are taken regularly

Patient instructions before and after the procedure

- ▶ Nothing by mouth for 12 hours before the examination.
- ▶ No solid foods for 30 minutes after the examination.
- ▶ Allow for aftereffects of sedation (no driving, no hazardous work activities for 24 hours).
- ▶ Report any complications (pain, bleeding, fever).

Risks and complications

- ▶ **Complication rate** of diagnostic endoscopy
  - – Overall complication rate $< 0.1\%$
  - – Mortality $< 0.01\%$
- ▶ **Cardiac** complications
  - – Ischemia, arrhythmias
- ▶ **Pulmonary** complications
  - – Hypoxia, aspiration
- ▶ **Bleeding and perforation**
- ▶ **Infection**
- ▶ Complications from **medications used during the procedure**
  - – Pharyngeal anesthesia: allergy, aspiration
  - – Sedation: respiratory depression, hypotension
- ▶ Complications of **therapeutic endoscopy** (sclerotherapy of esophageal varices, bougie or balloon dilation of the esophagus, polypectomy)
  - – Bleeding, perforation, mediastinitis, fistulation, pleural effusion
- ▶ Complications of **percutaneous endoscopic gastrostomy (PEG) placement** and **percutaneous endoscopic jejunostomy (PEJ) placement**
  - – Local infection, peritonitis, bleeding, sepsis

General

Preparations for Endoscopy: Medications (1)

■ Premedication and Medications Used During the Procedure

It is not strictly necessary to premedicate or medicate patients for upper GI endoscopy. The use and selection of medications should be tailored to the individual case. The following types of medication may be used:

▶ Local anesthetics
▶ Sedatives
▶ Analgesics
▶ Narcotics
▶ Antispasmodics
▶ Defoaming agents

Local Anesthesia

Indication

▶ Pharyngeal anesthesia can be used in any endoscopic procedure.

Contraindications

▶ Emergency endoscopy (increased risk of aspiration)
▶ Known hypersensitivity

Advantage

▶ Better patient tolerance of the examination

Disadvantages

▶ Increased risk of aspiration
▶ Allergic reaction
▶ Bad taste
▶ Cough
▶ Swallowing difficulties after the examination

Method

▶ Two squirts of lidocaine sprayed into the pharynx

Precautions

▶ Nothing by mouth from 30 minutes to one hour after the examination

Sedation

Indications

▶ Requested by the patient
▶ Very anxious patient

Contraindications

▶ Emergency endoscopy in a nonintubated patient
▶ Respiratory failure
▶ Circulatory failure

Advantages

▶ Improves subjective patient tolerance
▶ Makes examination easier to perform
▶ Suppresses sympathetic outflow
▶ Reduces hypertension, arrhythmias, coronary ischemia

Disadvantages

▶ Respiratory depression
▶ Less cooperative patient
▶ Paradoxical reaction
▶ Risk of aspiration

Method

▶ Goal is conscious sedation
▶ Midazolam (Dormicum), 2–5 (up to 10) mg i. v., half-life two to three hours
▶ Diazepam (Valium), 5–20 mg i. v., half-life 30 hours (!)

Precautions

▶ Close patient surveillance
▶ Pulse oximetry
▶ Intravenous line
▶ Have O_2 available
▶ Have antagonists available: flumazenil (Anexate)
▶ **Caution:** Midazolam has a longer half-life than flumazenil

Analgesia

Indications

▶ Indicated only for painful procedures
  – Bougie or balloon dilatation, PEG placement

Contraindications

▶ Emergency endoscopy in a nonintubated patient
▶ Respiratory failure
▶ Circulatory failure

Preparations for Endoscopy: Medications (2)

General

Analgesia (cont.)

Advantage

▶ Better tolerance of painful procedures

Disadvantages

▶ Respiratory depression
▶ Circulatory depression
▶ Bradycardia

Method

▶ Pethidine (Dolantin), 50–100 mg i. v.
▶ Piritramide (Dipidolor), 7.5–15 mg i. v.

Precautions

▶ Same as for benzodiazepines
▶ Have antagonists available: naloxone (Narcanti)

Antispasmodic

Indications

▶ Pyloric stenosis
▶ Duodenal biopsy
▶ Visualization of duodenal diverticula

Contraindications

▶ Note the contraindications for the agent used
▶ Butylscopolamine
  – Glaucoma, prostatic hypertrophy, arrhythmias

Advantage

▶ Eliminates possible interference from peristalsis

Disadvantage

▶ Side effects

Method

▶ Butylscopolamine, 5–20 mg i. v.

Precautions

▶ No special precautions are needed

Defoaming Agent

Indication

▶ Can be used in any endoscopic procedure

Contraindications

▶ None

Advantage

▶ Provides a clearer view in the stomach and duodenum

Disadvantage

▶ None

Method

▶ Several milliliters diluted with some water, administered orally just before the examination.
▶ In intubated patients, inject through the working channel, then flush (!) because the agent is sticky.

Precautions

▶ None

General Anesthesia

Indications

▶ Pediatric endoscopy
▶ Endoscopy in high-risk patients

Contraindication

▶ Age < three years

Advantages

▶ Better patient tolerance of the examination

Disadvantages

▶ Side effects
  – Fall in blood pressure, occasional rise in blood pressure, bradycardia, apnea, etc.

Agent

▶ Propofol (Diprivan)

Precautions

▶ Same as for sedation
▶ A second physician trained in emergency medicine should be in attendance

Checklists Before, During, and After the Examination

24 hours before the examination

- ☑ Confirm indication
- ☑ Check contraindications
- ☑ Necessary lab tests ordered? (blood count, coagulation)
- ☑ Antibiotic prophylaxis? (see p. 4)
- ☑ Informed consent obtained?
- ☑ Patient instructed about fasting?
- ☑ Cardiac pacemaker?
- ☑ Risk factors? (heart, lung, coagulation, general health)

Immediately before the examination

- ☑ Patient welcomed to the unit, greeted by name
- ☑ Signed consent form?
- ☑ Dentures removed?
- ☑ Defoaming agent administered?
- ☑ Coagulation tested?
- ☑ If necessary: peripheral venous access? (especially with sedation and for interventions)
- ☑ Equipment check? (air, suction)
- ☑ Endoscope tip lubricated
- ☑ Pharyngeal anesthesia (if desired)
- ☑ Contact with patient: "Here we go."

During the examination

- ☑ Talk to the patient, explain what is happening.
- ☑ Keep the patient in a left lateral position.
- ☑ Observe the patient (sweating, restlessness, facial expression, gestures, pain manifestations, breathing, skin color).
- ☑ If in doubt: pulse oximetry, echocardiogram (ECG) monitoring.

Diagnosis and Treatment of Complications (1)

The patient may develop or manifest complications during or immediately after the examination, or complications may arise after a complaint-free interval. They may involve the central nervous system, respiration, cardiovascular system, infections, allergic reactions, and of course the examined organs themselves: the pharynx, esophagus, stomach, and duodenum (see also Risks and Complications, p. 3, and Disclosure and Informed Consent, p. 8).

Immediate complications. The most frequent complaints and complications that occur during or immediately after the examination are as follows:
▶ Restlessness, agitation, pain, coughing, retching
▶ Dyspnea
▶ Apnea
▶ Loss of consciousness
▶ Bleeding

Delayed complications. The most frequent complaints and complications that arise after an initial complaint-free interval are as follows:
▶ Pain
▶ Dyspnea
▶ Signs of upper gastrointestinal bleeding: hematemesis, melena
▶ Signs of hypovolemic shock

Aid to decision-making. The tables below are designed to help with decision-making when complications arise. We cannot offer one standard protocol, especially for complaints that arise acutely during the examination. The decision must be made on a case-by-case basis, taking into account the patient's age and medical history, current status, and the clinical problem.

If in doubt, **withdraw the endoscope** because:
▶ The patient may actually be in danger.
▶ The patient should never be subjected to undue discomfort.
▶ In most cases, the instrument can be reinserted without difficulty.
▶ The instrument may become damaged. Always protect the endoscope with a bite guard!

■ Complications During the Examination

Restlessness, Agitation, Pain, Coughing, Gagging

Causes
▶ Normal response to the examination
▶ Faulty examination technique (especially, poor intubation technique)
▶ Not enough verbal reassurance, inadequate preparation for the procedure
▶ Misdirected intubation, retroflexion in the pharynx
▶ Pain due to unfavorable patient position
▶ Paradoxical reaction to sedation
▶ Respiratory distress, pain, angina pectoris
▶ Preexisting illness:
– Bronchial asthma, chronic obstructive lung disease
– Alcohol abuse
– Previous unpleasant endoscopy

Brief assessment
▶ Endoscope position (retroflexed? misdirected?)
▶ Verbal responsiveness of patient, cooperativeness
▶ O$_2$ saturation
▶ Heart rate

Reasons for stopping the examination and withdrawing the endoscope
▶ Serious preexisting illness
▶ Elderly patient
▶ Tachycardia > 140 bpm, arrhythmia
▶ O$_2$ saturation < 90 %, declining
▶ Uncooperative patient
▶ Angina pectoris

Reasons for pausing but leaving the instrument in place
▶ No preexisting illness
▶ Young patient
▶ O$_2$ saturation > 90 %
▶ Patient responsive to verbal commands
▶ Patient and endoscopist agree to continue

Treatment
▶ According to cause

Diagnosis and Treatment of Complications (2)

Dyspnea

Causes

- Psychogenic
- Obstructed nasal breathing
- Misdirected intubation, aspiration
- Bronchoconstriction, mucus congestion
- Cardiac decompensation

Brief assessment

- Respiratory rate, breath sound, cyanosis
- O_2 saturation
- Pulse

Reasons for stopping the examination and withdrawing the endoscope

- Elderly patient
- Preexisting cardiopulmonary disease
- O_2 saturation $< 90\%$, declining
- Tachycardia > 140 bpm

Reasons for pausing but leaving the instrument in place

- No preexisting illness
- Young patient
- Adequate O_2 saturation ($> 95\%$)

General treatment

- For significant dyspnea, treat according to the general rules for cardiopulmonary resuscitation:
- A Clear the airway and keep it open (suction out mucus, vomitus, etc.).
- B Ventilate (O_2 by mask or nasal catheter); intubate if response is poor.
- C Maintain and stabilize the circulation, if necessary using external cardiac massage.
- D Place an intravenous line, give specific pharmacotherapy.

Specific treatments

- For **bronchoconstriction**
  - Theophylline, 200 mg i. v.
  - Prednisolone, 100 mg i. v.
  - Beta-2 mimetics by aerosol
  - Beta-2 mimetics s.c. (e.g., Bricanyl 0.5–1.0 mg s.c.)
- For **cardiac decompensation**
  - Nitroglycerine subl.
  - Furosemide, 40–80 mg i. v.
  - With concomitant bronchospasm: theophylline, 200 mg i. v.
  - Treatment of cardiac arrhythmias

Apnea

Causes

- Pharmacological: sedation, analgesia
- Cardiac: asystole, ventricular fibrillation, bradycardia
- Anaphylactic shock

Course of action

- Discontinue examination, withdraw endoscope

Brief assessment

- Respiratory excursions, O_2 saturation
- Carotid pulse

General treatment

- Follow the general rules for cardiopulmonary resuscitation:
- A Clear the airway and keep it open (suction out mucus, vomitus, etc.).
- B Ventilate (O_2 by mask or nasal catheter); intubate if response is poor.
- C Maintain and stabilize the circulation, if necessary using external cardiac massage.
- D Place an intravenous line, give specific pharmacotherapy.

Specific treatments

- For antagonizing the effect of **benzodiazepines**
  - Flumazenil (Anexate), 0.5–1 mg i. v., repeat after three minutes if necessary
  - Caution: half-life of flumazenil $<$ half-life of midazolam $<<$ half-life of diazepam
- For antagonizing the effect of **opiates**
  - Naloxone (Narcanti), 0.4–2 mg, repeat after three minutes if necessary
- For a **cardiac cause**
  - Bradycardia: 0.5–1 mg atropine i. v., may require temporary pacemaker
  - Asystole: precordial thump, 0.5–1 mg epinephrine in 10 mL NaCl i. v., temporary pacemaker
  - Ventricular fibrillation: cardioversion (200, 300, 360 J), repeat after 1 mg epinephrine in 10 mL NaCl i. v.
- For **anaphylaxis**
  - Epinephrine, 0.25–0.5 mg in 10 mL NaCl i. v.
  - Prednisolone, 250 mg i. v.
  - Antihistamine (e.g., 2 mg clemastine i. v.)
  - Volume: 500–1000 mL (e.g., crystalline or colloidal plasma substitute)

1

Diagnosis and Treatment of Complications (3)

General

Loss of Consciousness

Causes

▶ Sedation or analgesia
▶ Hypoxia
▶ Asystole or ventricular fibrillation
▶ Anaphylaxis

Course of action

▶ Discontinue examination, withdraw instrument

Brief assessment

▶ Verbal responsiveness, response to painful stimuli
▶ Respiratory excursions, O_2 saturation
▶ Carotid pulse

General treatment

▶ Follow the general rules for cardiopulmonary resuscitation:
A Clear the airway and keep it open (suction out mucus, vomitus, etc.).
B Ventilate (O_2 by mask or nasal catheter); intubate if response is poor.
C Maintain and stabilize the circulation, if necessary using external cardiac massage.
D Place an intravenous line, give specific pharmacotherapy.

Specific treatments

▶ Antagonize effects of benzodiazepines (see Apnea, p. 13).
▶ Antagonize effects of opiates (see Apnea, p. 13).
▶ Treat a cardiac cause (see Apnea, p. 13).
▶ Treat for anaphylaxis (see Apnea, p. 13).

Bleeding

Causes

▶ Instrument tip contact (pharynx, upper esophageal sphincter, duodenal bulb)
▶ Varices (ulcerations in the esophagus, stomach, and duodenum)
▶ Mallory–Weiss syndrome
▶ Less common causes (see p. 155)
▶ Coagulation disorders, thrombocytopenia

Course of action

▶ Do not withdraw the endoscope!

Treatment

▶ Treat for upper gastrointestinal bleeding (see p. 146)

■ Complications Immediately after the Examination or after a Complaint-Free Interval

Pain

Causes

▶ Neck: pharyngeal injury, esophageal perforation
▶ Chest: esophageal perforation, angina pectoris
▶ Abdomen: overdistension, perforation of the stomach or duodenum

Diagnosis

▶ Clinical findings
  – Pharyngeal inspection, cutaneous emphysema, abdominal findings

▶ Radiographic findings
  – Plain film of the neck and chest (cutaneous emphysema? air in mediastinum?)
  – Standing abdominal plain film (free air?)
  – Abdominal plain film in LLD (free air?)
▶ ECG if a cardiac cause is suspected

Treatment

▶ NPO
▶ Further treatment according to cause (see below)

Diagnosis and Treatment of Complications (4)

Esophageal Perforation

Risk factors
- Uncooperative patient
- Diverticula (especially Zenker diverticula), strictures, ulcers
- Osteophytes
- Interventions
- Bougie or balloon dilation, sclerotherapy of varices

Symptoms
- Pain (neck, chest, back)
- Cutaneous emphysema
- Dysphagia

Diagnosis
- Radiographic findings
  - Plain film of chest and neck (free air?)
  - Contrast examination of the esophagus (with water-soluble medium)

Treatment
- Surgical treatment
- Conservative treatment only in selected cases
- NPO
- Antibiotics, proton pump inhibitor (PPI) i. v.

Perforation of the Stomach or Duodenum

Risk factors
- Duodenal diverticula
- Interventions (polypectomy, laser therapy)

Symptoms
- Pain (epigastric, diffuse), peritonism
- Diminished bowel sounds
- Fall in blood pressure, tachycardia, sweating
- Fever

Diagnosis
- Radiographic findings
  - Standing abdominal plain film (free air?)
  - Abdominal plain film in LLD (free air?)

Treatment
- Surgical treatment
- Conservative treatment only in selected cases
- NPO, nasogastric tube
- Antibiotics, PPI

Pharyngeal Injury
- Otolaryngological diagnosis and treatment

Myocardial Ischemia
- Diagnosis and treatment according to established guidelines

Dyspnea

Causes
- Aspiration
- Cardiac decompensation

Symptoms
- Tachypnea? Cyanosis? Tachycardia?

Diagnosis
- Auscultation
- Arterial blood gas analysis
- Chest radiograph
- ECG

Treatment
- According to cause (see below)

Diagnosis and Treatment of Complications (5)

Aspiration or Aspiration Pneumonia

Risk factors

- ▶ Sedation, pharyngeal anesthesia
- ▶ Uncooperative patients, elderly patients
- ▶ Patients with swallowing difficulties, with multiple morbidity
- ▶ Emergency endoscopy

Symptoms

- ▶ Dyspnea, cyanosis
- ▶ Tachycardia, fever

Diagnosis

- ▶ Auscultation
  - – Fine or coarse rales
- ▶ Radiographs
  - – May be negative initially (!), diffuse patchy infiltration

Treatment

- ▶ Antibiotics (e.g., cefoxitin, tobramycin)
- ▶ Prednisolone, 250 mg i. v.
- ▶ O_2 by nasal catheter; if no response, intubate and ventilate

Complications

- ▶ Global respiratory failure
- ▶ Adult respiratory distress syndrome (ARDS)
- ▶ Abscess

Cardiac Decompensation

Risk factors

- ▶ Elderly patients
- ▶ Preexisting cardiovascular disease
- ▶ Anemia

Symptoms

- ▶ Dyspnea, tachycardia, frothy sputum
- ▶ Acrocyanosis
- ▶ Cold sweats

Diagnosis

- ▶ Auscultation
  - – Sometimes normal (!); moist rales, bronchospasm
- ▶ Radiographic findings
  - – Symmetrical hilar shadow, cardiac enlargement, Kerley B lines
- ▶ ECG
  - – Ischemia? Arrhythmias?

Treatment

- ▶ O_2 by nasal catheter
- ▶ Nitrates, furosemide
- ▶ Treatment of arrhythmia
- ▶ Antiangina therapy as required

Hematemesis, Melena, Hypovolemia

Risk factors

- ▶ Varices
- ▶ Gastric and duodenal ulcer
- ▶ Thrombopenia, coagulation disorders, anticoagulant therapy
- ▶ Interventions (polypectomy, mucosectomy)

Symptoms

- ▶ Hematemesis
- ▶ Melena
- ▶ Symptoms of hemorrhagic shock

Diagnosis

- ▶ Endoscopy

Treatment

- ▶ See relevant chapters.

Endoscopic Technique: Steps in Learning

■ Learning the Examination Technique

Endoscopy training proceeds in a series of steps (Table 1.7):

The first step is familiarization with the endoscope—learning how to handle the instrument properly and how to operate the valves and control wheels. The trainee performs "dry runs" to practice manipulating the instrument shaft and controls: push, pull, rotation, up/down angulation, and right/left angulation.

In the second step, the trainee assists an experienced endoscopist. The instructor passes and directs the endoscope and gives instructions. The trainee pulls and advances the endoscope and observes the procedure through a teaching attachment or on the video monitor. In this way the novice gains a feel for the effects of pushing and pulling the instrument.

In the third step, the trainee takes over the endoscope after it has been positioned loosely in the duodenum and inspects the duodenal lumen during withdrawal while the instructor pulls back the endoscope. This is a relatively safe way to give the trainee a feel for manipulating the controls. The trainee learns how to obtain a luminal view and keep the lumen centered in the image while the instrument is being withdrawn. This step often involves the first disappointment, as many beginners will find it surprisingly difficult to keep the lumen centered in the image.

In the fourth step, the trainee introduces the endoscope and conducts the examination under the direct supervision of the instructor, who does the actual pushing of the instrument while monitoring the procedure.

In the fifth step the trainee performs an examination solo, but the instructor is ready to step in if problems arise.

■ Handling the Endoscope

The control head of the endoscope is held in the left hand. The index and middle fingers activate the suction and air/water valves. Many examiners operate the angulation control wheels with the right hand, but an endoscopist with large hands can also manage these controls with the left hand. This leaves the right hand free to manipulate the insertion tube, which is advantageous in some situations. The control head is used to control the four functional systems listed in Table 1.8.

Optics

In a conventional endoscope, the control head has an eyepiece that allows for individual focusing. A video endoscope dispenses with this function, transmitting the image electronically from a distal chip to a video monitor.

The endoscopist should rehearse instrument manipulations to get a feel for how the image is transmitted from object to eyepiece. When the endoscope shaft is in a straightened position, it gives an upright view of the object with the right and left sides correctly displayed. Bending the shaft in the 12/6-o'clock plane correctly displays the right and left sides but inverts the image by 180°. Bending in the 3/9-o'clock plane results in an upright image with the left and right sides reversed.

Table 1.7 **Five-step program for endoscopy training**

1. Bench practice with the endoscope.
2. The instructor controls the endoscope while the trainee pushes the shaft and watches the procedure using a teaching attachment or video monitor.
3. The instructor advances the instrument, the trainee withdraws it.
4. The trainee advances and withdraws the instrument under supervision.
5. Solo endoscopy by the trainee.

Table 1.8 **Control head functions**

▶ Eyepiece or video output
▶ Tip angulation controls
▶ Air insufflation/irrigation
▶ Suction/instrumentation

Endoscopic Technique: Maneuvering the Scope

Fig. 1.**6 Effect of straightening the endoscope**

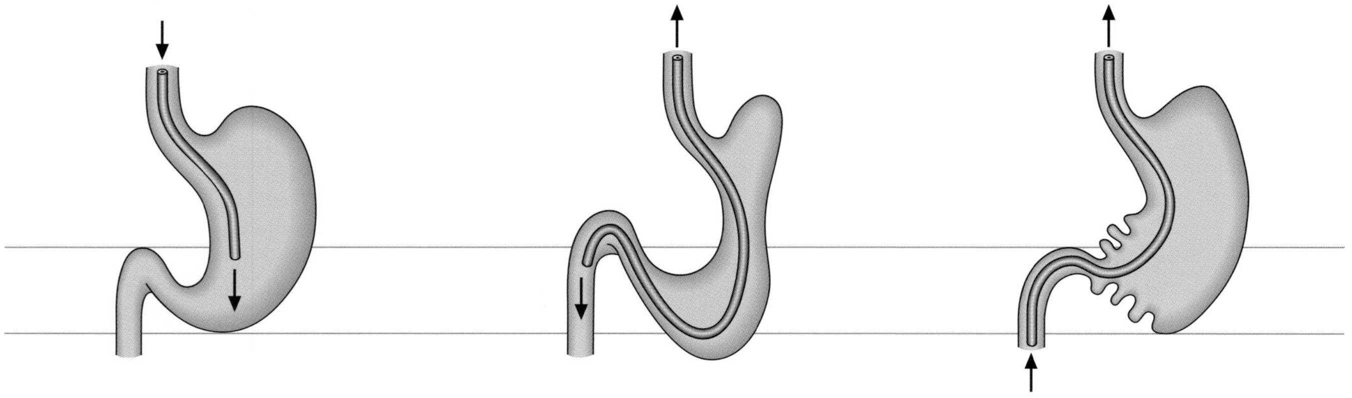

a Pushing the instrument forward initially causes it to advance. On reaching the antrum, the endoscope tends to slacken and form a large loop in the stomach

b The angled endoscope tip is in the duodenum. Pulling back on the shaft will straighten the loop in the stomach, causing the tip to advance down the duodenum

c When the loop has been completely straightened, further pulling will effect a withdrawal of the endoscope tip

Fig. 1.**7 Rotation.** Effect of a rotating movement on a bowed endoscope

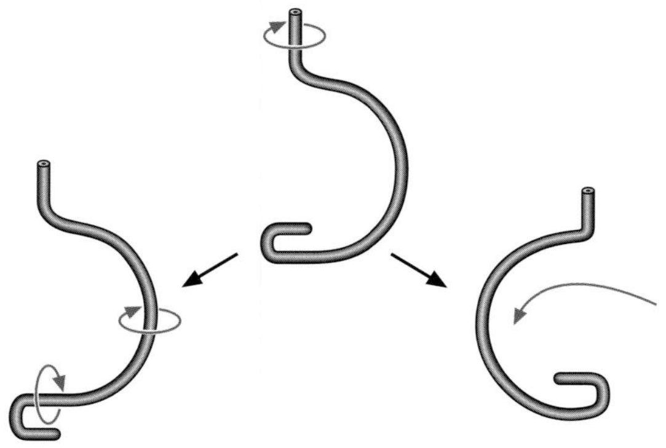

a When the bow is defined by the shape of the lumen

b When the endoscope is free to move

Table 1.9   **The elements of endoscope movements**

▶ Angulation
▶ Push/pull
▶ Rotation
▶ Bowing

Mechanics of Endoscope Movements

The individual components of endoscope movements are listed in Table 1.**9**.

Angulation

The bending section of the endoscope is controlled with two angulation wheels, which deflect the tip by means of pull wires. The large inner wheel moves the endoscope tip up and down, and the smaller outer wheel deflects it to the left and right (in the 3/9-o'clock plane).

Pushing and Pulling

The fact that the endoscope can be advanced and withdrawn is self-evident. It should be noted, however, that when the instrument tip is retroflexed into a "J" shape, pulling back on the endoscope will advance the tip toward the object being viewed.

Moreover, when the endoscope is bowed into a large loop, pulling back on the instrument will straighten the shaft, initially causing the endoscope tip to advance by several centimeters. This phenomenon occurs routinely in the proximal duodenum (Fig. 1.**6**).

Rotation

Rotation of the endoscope about its long axis is transmitted to the tip of the torque–stable shaft, virtually without spiral twisting. Thus, when the instrument tip is in a raised position, the shaft can be rotated as an alternative to using the right/left control wheel.

Bowing/Looping

Passive bowing or looping of the endoscope is determined by the anatomical shape of the lumen that surrounds the shaft. Though not actively controlled by the endoscopist, it is always an element of instrument control. This is because the actual effect of a rotating maneuver depends on the overall bend of the endoscope, on the freedom of movement of the endoscope within the organ and of the organ itself, and on the position of the bending section (Fig. 1.**7**).

Overall Control

The application of these control maneuvers cannot be learned theoretically. Endoscopic control is a very complex process whose separate elements are not always precisely known. The overall effect of combined control maneuvers can be learned only through practice.

Endoscopic Technique: Functions

Air Insufflation and Irrigation

The light source is combined with a compressed air pump that can deliver either compressed air or pressurized water through the umbilical cord to the endoscope, as desired. This function is controlled by the air/water valve. This valve has three positions (Fig. 1.**8**):

▶ Neutral position: no air insufflation, no water jet
▶ Air insufflation
▶ Irrigation (water jet)

Fig. 1.8 Air insufflation and irrigation

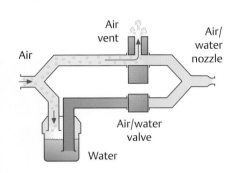 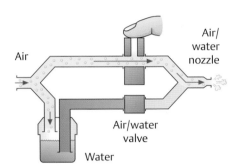 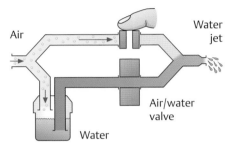

a Air/water valve in the neutral position. The air/water valve permits air to exit through a vent hole. The vented air can be felt by holding a finger over the hole. When this valve is not activated, it automatically assumes a position that blocks the water channel while allowing air to escape through the vent hole

b Air insufflation. Placing the finger lightly on the vent hole keeps the air from escaping and redirects it to the distal end of the endoscope. This does not involve activating the valve

c Irrigation. Pressing the valve button down closes off the air channel and redirects air pressure into the water bottle, causing water to be pumped from the bottle into the endoscope. The air and water channels converge at the distal end of the scope and open at the air/water nozzle

---

Suction and Instrumentation

The suction channel and instrument channel converge at the distal end of the control head to a common channel that passes down the shaft to the suction/instrument channel opening at the distal bending section. The tapered connector for the suction pump tube is located on the side of the supply plug. Suction is controlled by the suction valve on the control head, which has two positions (Fig. 1.**9**):

▶ Neutral position
▶ Suction position

Fig. 1.9 Suction and instrumentation

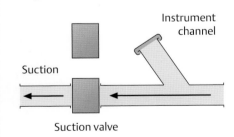 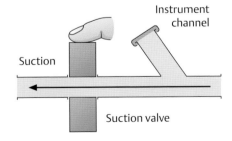 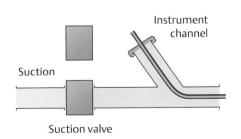

a Suction valve in the neutral position. When the suction valve is not activated, it automatically assumes the neutral position and blocks suction

b Suction position. Pushing the valve button opens the suction channel, creating a negative pressure that draws air or fluid into the opening of the suction/instrument channel at the distal end of the scope. Because the proximal opening of the instrument channel communicates with the suction channel, this opening must be occluded with a valve

c Instrumentation. Instruments (injection needles, biopsy forceps, catheters) can be introduced through the instrument channel and passed down the endoscope. The instrument channel can be used to flush the suction channel if the latter becomes clogged, and it can be used for introducing large amounts of fluid (e.g., to irrigate a bleeding lesion)

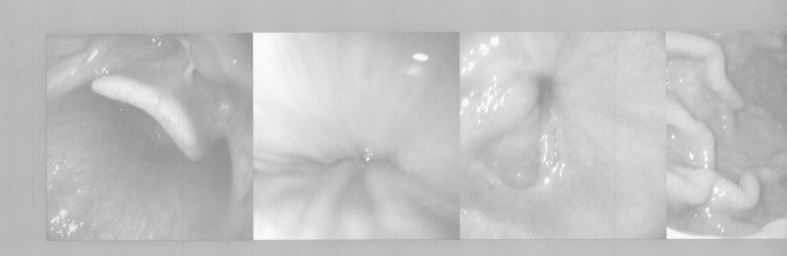

2 Examination Technique and Normal Findings

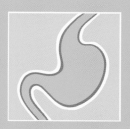

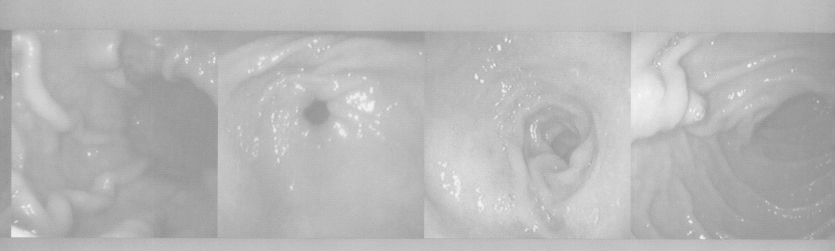

Inserting the Endoscope

■ Basic Rules

Several methods can be used to insert the endoscope. None of these methods has major advantages over the others, but certain rules need to be followed (Fig. 2.1). Because insertion of the endoscope is the most unpleasant part of the examination for most patients, it should be carried out in a calm, assured manner. The patient lies on the left side with the chin tucked against the chest. The bite guard may be placed securely between the teeth at this time, or it may be fitted over the instrument shaft before sliding the endoscope carefully into the mouth. In the latter case, the bite guard is not placed until the endoscope has entered the upper esophagus. If difficulties arise, especially due to interference from the tongue, the fingers can be used to assist endoscope insertion. In rare cases the patient may have difficulty tolerating the procedure in left lateral decubitus, and the endoscopist may attempt to pass the scope with the patient sitting up. This should be reserved for exceptional cases, however.

Fig.2.**1 Inserting the endoscope**

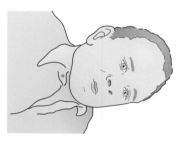

a The patient is in the left lateral position

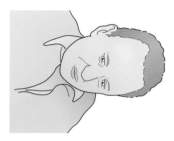

b The chin is tucked against the chest

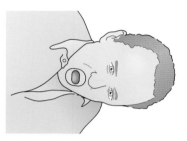

c The bite guard is placed

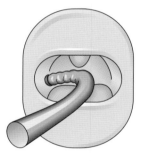

d The endoscope tip is preangled and inserted through the bite guard

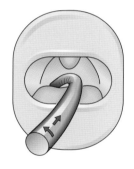

e Once inside the mouth, the slightly angled endoscope tip is rotated into the mesopharynx and advanced

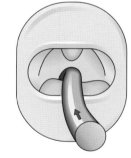

f The endoscope is advanced toward the hypopharynx

Alternative method

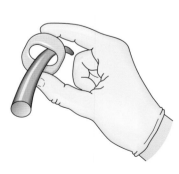

g The bite guard is fitted over the instrument shaft

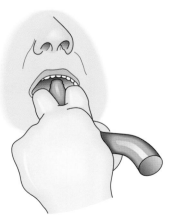

h Insertion is aided by guiding the endoscope tip with the index and middle fingers

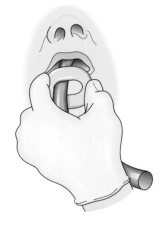

i After the endoscope is in the hypopharynx, the bite guard is slid into place

Blind Insertion

■ With Visual Control

In the blind insertion method, the endoscope is first passed over the base of the tongue toward the hypopharynx under external visual control. Care is taken that the endoscope tip is not retroflexed toward the nasopharynx and does not deviate to the left or right into the piriform recess (Figs. 2.**2**, 2.**3**). With proper technique, the instrument tip can be advanced just to the introitus of the upper esophageal sphincter, at which time the patient is instructed to swallow.

■ Passage through the Upper Esophageal Sphincter

Unless the patient swallows, it is extremely difficult to advance the endoscope through the upper esophageal sphincter without causing injury or significant discomfort. Endoscope insertion is contraindicated while the patient is coughing or taking a deep breath, as this will inevitably lead to tracheal intubation (Fig. 2.**2**). The period immediately after coughing, when the patient is swallowing saliva, is a favorable time for entering the esophagus. At this time the larynx is in an elevated position, visible externally on the neck. The endoscope is advanced by applying gentle pressure. Following initial resistance, a distinct "give" is felt as the endoscope slips into the upper esophagus. Once the instrument tip is within the esophagus, the insertion is continued under endoscopic vision.

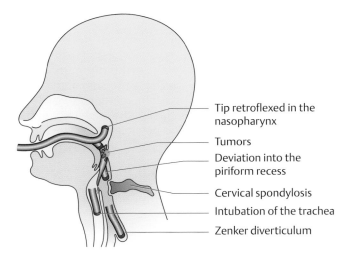

Tip retroflexed in the nasopharynx

Tumors

Deviation into the piriform recess

Cervical spondylosis

Intubation of the trachea

Zenker diverticulum

Fig. 2.**2**   **Risks and hazards of endoscope insertion**

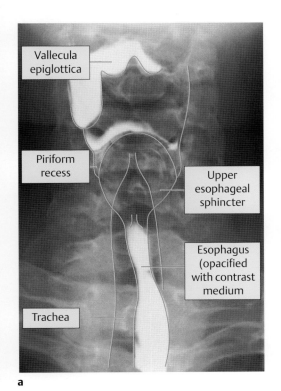

Vallecula epiglottica

Piriform recess

Upper esophageal sphincter

Esophagus (opacified with contrast medium

Trachea

a

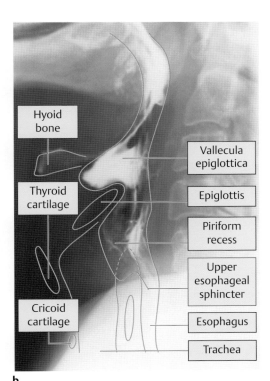

Hyoid bone

Vallecula epiglottica

Thyroid cartilage

Epiglottis

Piriform recess

Upper esophageal sphincter

Cricoid cartilage

Esophagus

Trachea

b

Fig. 2.**3**   **Larynx and pharynx**
a   Anteroposterior (AP) radiograph after oral contrast administration. The piriform recess descends lateral to the larynx. Medial to it is the introitus of the upper esophageal sphincter
b   Lateral radiograph after oral contrast administration. The piriform recess appears as an outpouching structure lateral and anterior to the upper esophageal sphincter

2

Direct-Vision Insertion

Esophageal intubation can also be performed under direct endoscopic vision (Fig. 2.**6**). The instrument tip is advanced to the larynx as described above. The open glottic aperture is seen (Fig. 2.**4**). A slit can be identified between the posterior wall of the hypopharynx and the cuneiform and corniculate tubercles, which are clearly visible in most patients. This slit (not shown in this view) leads to the upper esophageal sphincter, which curves gently around the posterior side of the cricoid cartilage. The posterior wall of the larynx bulges far into the hypopharynx, making central passage difficult. The instrument tip should pass a little to the left or right of the midline, taking care not to deviate into either piriform recess. The instrument is advanced with gentle pressure until the patient swallows. The esophageal lumen becomes visible for a brief moment, and the tip is advanced into the esophagus. In many cases it is also possible to position the endoscope carefully at the esophageal introitus, have the patient swallow several times, and rotate the instrument into the esophagus. Care is taken not to slip into the piriform recess (Fig. 2.**6**).

■ Problems

▶ In both methods—blind and direct-vision insertion—there is always a short segment of the esophagus that must be traversed without vision.
▶ If a Zenker diverticulum is present in this region, there is a substantial risk of perforation.
▶ If the endoscope is misdirected toward the trachea, the vocal cords (Fig. 2.**5a**) or the typical ribbed walls of the trachea (Fig. 2.**5b**) will be seen. In this case the endoscope should be withdrawn at once.

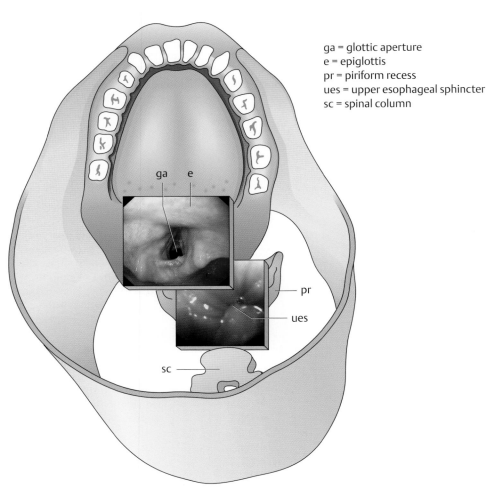

ga = glottic aperture
e = epiglottis
pr = piriform recess
ues = upper esophageal sphincter
sc = spinal column

Fig. 2.**4** **View of the trachea and upper esophageal sphincter.** Notice that the slitlike upper esophageal sphincter, not yet visible in the upper plane, lies between the interarytenoid incisure and the spinal column. The epiglottis, which extends to a relatively high level, is usually difficult to identify. The lower plane is at the level of the upper esophageal sphincter

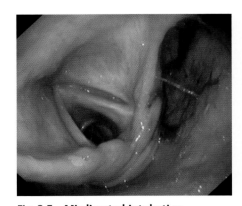

Fig. 2.**5** **Misdirected intubation**
a Impending tracheal intubation. View of the vocal cords

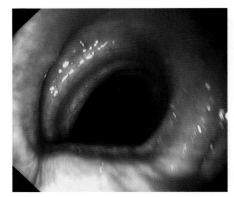

b The typical ridged contours of the trachea can be seen

Direct-Vision Insertion: Four Phases

Fig. 2.**6 Intubation of the esophagus**

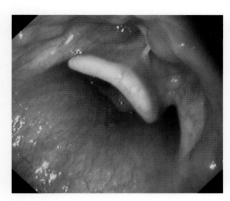 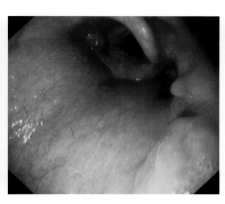 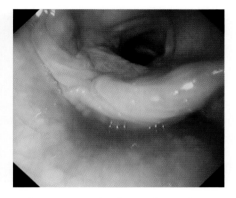

a The instrument tip is over the base of the tongue. The upper border of the epiglottis is visible

b The instrument has been advanced. View into the hypopharynx

c The instrument has been advanced further. The esophageal inlet is visible at the 6-o'clock position

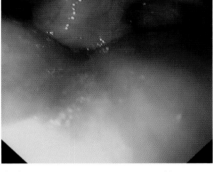

d The instrument tip is positioned between the posterior wall of the hypopharynx and the posterior wall of the larynx. When the patient swallows, the upper esophageal sphincter can be seen

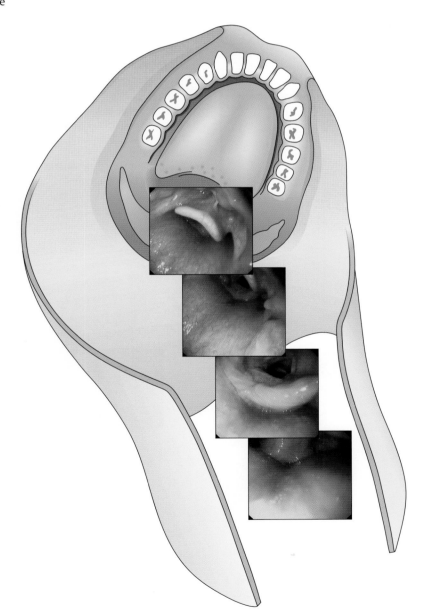

2

Upper Esophageal Sphincter

■ Anatomy

The esophagus is 20–24 cm long. It begins approximately 14–16 cm distal to the incisor teeth with the upper esophageal sphincter (Fig. 2.**8**) at the level of the cricoid cartilage and reaches the stomach at 38–41 cm.

■ Physiology

The upper esophageal sphincter forms the entrance to the esophagus. As the narrowest part of the alimentary tract, it is the first and often the most difficult obstacle for the endoscopist to surmount (Fig. 2.**7**). It is a muscular sphincter formed predominantly by the cricopharyngeal fibers of the constrictor pharyngeus muscle. This region forms a high-pressure zone 2–4 cm long with a resting pressure of 40–120 mmHg, making it extremely difficult to intubate. This pressure falls when the patient swallows, allowing the endoscope to pass through. The sphincter almost never has a visible lumen, since the relaxation phase during swallowing lasts for only a fraction of a second (Table 2.**1**).

Endoscopically, the upper esophageal sphincter appears as a lip-shaped eminence surrounding a transversely oriented, slitlike lumen (Figs. 2.**7**, 2.**9**). The stratified squamous epithelium of the esophagus itself normally appears reddish–gray with a smooth, glistening surface. It is not very transparent, but longitudinal, superficially branched venous plexuses can be seen beneath the mucosa.

Table 2.**1** **Upper esophageal sphincter**

▶ Approximately 14 cm from the incisor teeth
▶ Slitlike lumen
▶ Difficult to see into the lumen
▶ Endoscope can be passed only during swallowing
▶ **Caution:** Avoid slipping into the piriform recess.

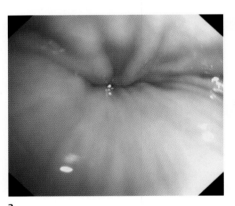

a

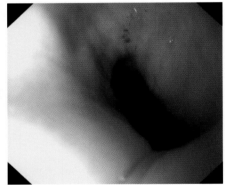

b

Fig. 2.**7** **Upper esophageal sphincter.** The tip of the endoscope is positioned directly above the upper esophageal sphincter
a The patient is breathing, and the esophageal sphincter is closed
b The patient swallows, and the esophageal sphincter briefly opens

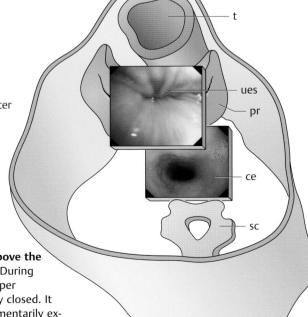

t = trachea
ues = upper esophageal sphincter
pr = piriform recess
ce = cervical esophagus
sc = spinal column

Fig. 2.**9** **Cross section just above the upper esophageal sphincter**. During esophageal intubation, the upper esophageal sphincter is usually closed. It opens during swallowing, momentarily exposing the lumen. At that time the endoscope can be advanced

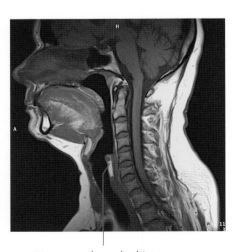

Upper esophageal sphincter

Fig. 2.**8** **Midsagittal scan through the head and neck** (from: Möller and Reif, *Normal Findings in CT and MRI*. Stuttgart: Thieme 1999)

Cervical Esophagus

■ Anatomy

The cervical esophagus begins just below the upper esophageal sphincter and is 6 cm long.

> Its distal end cannot be positively identified at endoscopy, however. The cervical esophagus is a straight, collapsed tube that appears largely featureless at endoscopy. Air insufflation distends it to a round, symmetrical lumen that is affected very little by respiratory movements (Figs. 2.**10**, 2.**11**; Table 2.**2**). The middle esophageal constriction is located approximately 27 cm from the incisor teeth, several centimeters past the junction with the thoracic esophagus.

Table 2.**2**   **Cervical esophagus**

▶ Approximately 16–20 cm from the incisor teeth
▶ Collapsed
▶ Symmetrical
▶ Round
▶ Delicate folds
▶ Straight course

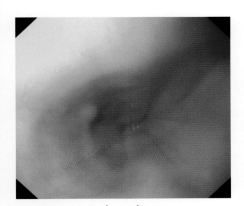

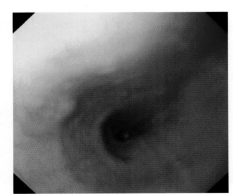

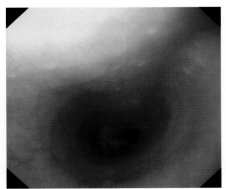

Fig. 2.10   Cervical esophagus
a Without air insufflation, the cervical esophagus is collapsed

b Slight air insufflation

c More forceful insufflation distends the esophagus, and the lumen appears round and symmetrical

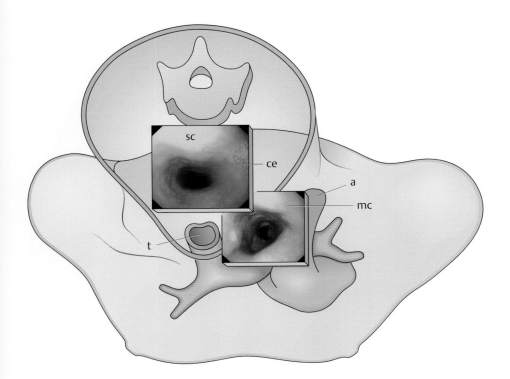

Fig. 2.11   Cross section at the level of the cervical esophagus. The cervical esophagus appears almost featureless at endoscopy. The next visible landmark is the midesophageal constriction
sc = spinal column
ce = cervical esophagus
a = aorta
mc = midesophageal constriction
t = trachea

Middle Esophageal Constriction

■ Anatomy

The middle esophageal constriction is reached at approximately 27 cm. It is the first definite landmark that is seen in passing through the otherwise featureless cervical and upper thoracic esophagus. It is an asymmetrical luminal constriction caused by indentations from the aorta and left main bronchus (Table 2.3).

The aorta and bronchus are difficult to identify as such in the endoscopic image, and it can be difficult to appreciate their spatial relationships. It is necessary to know the anatomy of this region and the orientation of the endoscope (Figs. 2.12, 2.13).

The aorta indents the esophagus from the lateral side and runs almost horizontally as it crosses the esophagus (Fig. 2.14a). The left main bronchus indents the esophagus from the anterior side. In the endoscopic image, it runs obliquely downward in a counterclockwise direction (Fig. 2.14b, c). It has a slightly ribbed surface. A posterior indentation from the spinal column is often seen opposite the bronchus. The aorta and bronchus cannot always be positively identified. Bizarre shapes are sometimes noted in thin patients.

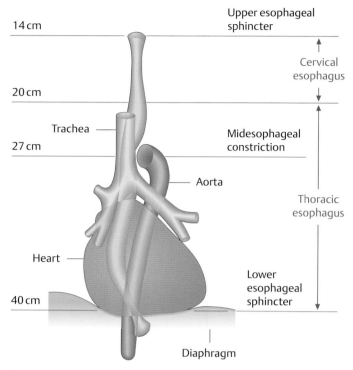

Fig. 2.**12** **Midesophageal constriction.** Standard anatomical view from the anterior aspect

Table 2.**3** **Midesophageal constriction**

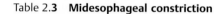

▶ Approximately 27 cm from the incisor teeth
▶ Indented by the aorta
▶ Indented by the left main bronchus

Fig. 2.**13** **Cross section at the level of the midesophageal constriction.** To understand the appearance of the midesophageal constriction in the upper image, it is necessary to know the rotational position of the endoscope. In this figure the indentation from the spinal column is approximately at the 12-o'clock position. The left main bronchus is at the 6-o'clock position, and the aortic arch is on the right. Notice that the aortic arch is more proximal than the bronchus and runs almost horizontally. The left main bronchus is distal and runs counterclockwise down below the aortic arch

a = aorta
re = retrocardial esophagus
l mb = left main bronchus
r mb = right main bronchus

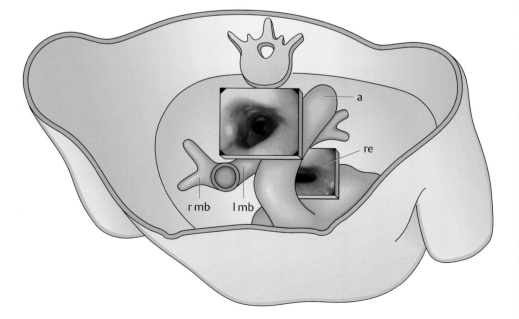

Inspecting the Middle Esophageal Constriction

Fig. 2.**14 Cross sections**

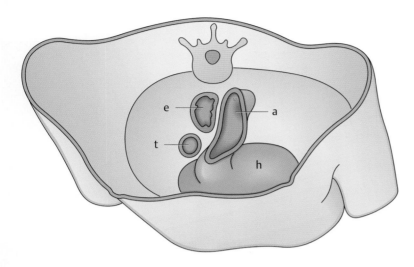

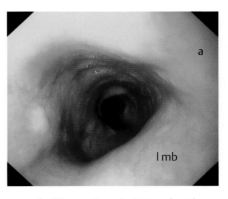

a Level of the aortic arch. Notice that this section is still proximal to the tracheal bifurcation, and the esophagus is indented only from the side by the aortic arch. The impression from the left main bronchus is seen distally in the endoscopic image

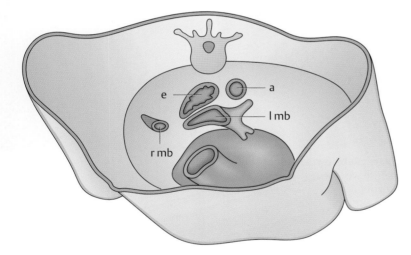

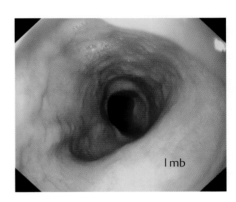

b Level of the left main bronchus. Notice that this section is just below the aortic arch. The esophagus is indented by the left main bronchus at this level

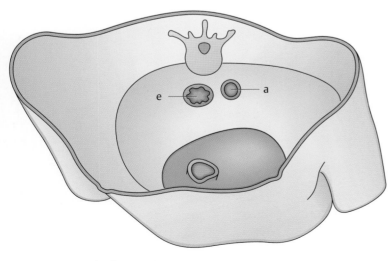

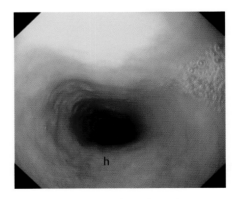

c Below the left main bronchus. The esophagus is indented only by the spinal column at the level of the cross section. The cardiac impression is seen distally in the image

e = esophagus	h = heart
a = aorta	l mb = left main bronchus
t = trachea	r mb = right main bronchus

Retrocardiac Esophagus

■ Anatomy

The retrocardiac esophagus begins approximately 30–38 cm from the incisor teeth. It is curved posteriorly at this level due to displacement by the heart (Fig. 2.15; Table 2.4).

The retrocardiac esophagus is visualized just below the middle esophageal constriction. This portion of the esophagus is compressed anteriorly by the left atrium and posteriorly by the aorta for a length of 8 cm, resulting in an elliptical lumen (Figs. 2.16, 2.17). Distinct pulsations can be seen.

Table 2.4 Retrocardiac esophagus

- ▶ Approximately 30–38 cm from the incisor teeth
- ▶ Elliptical indentation from the heart and aorta
- ▶ Bowed posteriorly, then curves forward toward the diaphragm
- ▶ Pulsations

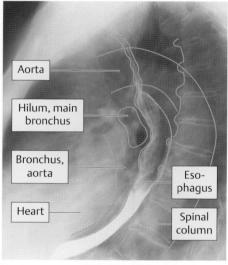

Fig. 2.15 Lateral chest radiograph after oral contrast administration. Midsagittal view of the retrocardiac esophagus. Notice that the entire esophagus is bowed posteriorly and is indented from the front by the heart

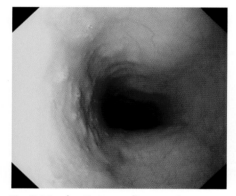 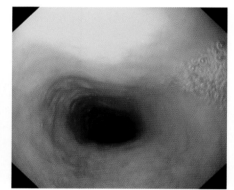

Fig. 2.16 a, b Retrocardiac esophagus. This region shows pulsatile changes in luminal shape   b

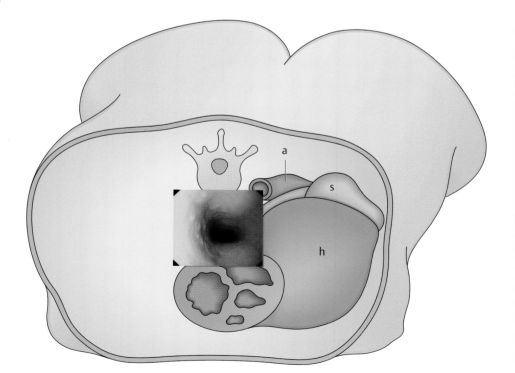

Fig. 2.17 Retrocardiac esophagus in cross section. Notice that the esophagus is symmetrically indented from the anterior side. The descending aorta is posterolateral to the esophagus
a = aorta
s = stomach
h = heart

Distal Esophagus and Lower Esophageal Constriction

■ Anatomy

The lower esophageal constriction is formed by a combination of the lower esophageal sphincter and extrinsic pressure from the diaphragmatic hiatus. It is reached at approximately 36–38 cm from the incisor teeth (Table 2.5).

> The lumen of the distal esophagus again appears round and symmetrical. The lower esophageal constriction is visible in the distance (Fig. 2.18). The muscular contraction and accompanying venous plexus create a typical endoscopic picture of longitudinal folds with concentric luminal narrowing (Fig. 2.19).

Table 2.5 **Lower esophageal constriction**

▶ Approximately 36–38 cm from the incisor teeth
▶ Formed by the sphincter and esophageal hiatus
▶ Venous plexus
▶ Longitudinal folds with concentric luminal narrowing

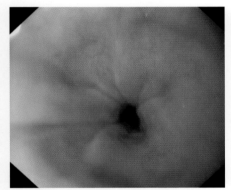 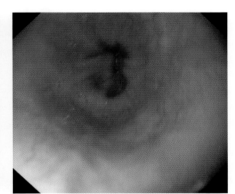

Fig. 2.18 a, b **Distal esophagus.** Views of the lower esophageal constriction

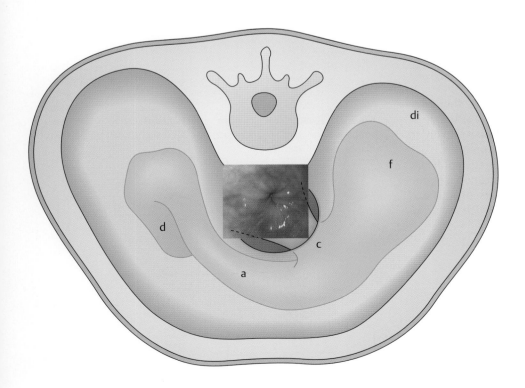

Fig. 2.19 **Cross section** just above the lower esophageal constriction
di = diaphragm
f = fundus
c = cardia
a = antrum
d = duodenum

Gastroesophageal Junction

■ Anatomy

The gastroesophageal junction is reached at approximately 38 (35–41) cm from the incisors. Besides the indentations from the aorta, left main bronchus, and heart, which give the esophagus a somewhat more variegated appearance, the gastroesophageal junction is the first truly interesting station that is reached during upper endoscopy. On the one hand, the gastroesophageal junction is a functionally and anatomically complex region that is not easily understood or evaluated (Fig. 2.**20**). At the same time, this region is one of the most frequent indications for upper GI endoscopy and is the site of the most common disease of the esophagus and of the upper gastrointestinal tract in general: reflux disease.

■ Physiology

The frequency of diseases and complaints in this region is understandable when we consider the stresses that exist there even under physiological conditions. The thoracic cavity is under a negative pressure that is maximal during inspiration. Meanwhile, the flattening of the diaphragm that occurs with inspiration causes a rise in intraabdominal pressure, which is maximal during coughing and straining. This results in a pressure gradient of 10–15 mmHg, which the organ structures in this region must be able to withstand. Additionally, the gastroesophageal junction marks the boundary between the acid-sensitive epithelium of the esophagus and the strongly acidic gastric contents. A technically complex apparatus is needed to handle the pressure gradient and pH differences that exist in this region

■ Closure Mechanisms

Three anatomical factors maintain the integrity of the gastroesophageal junction (Fig. 2.**21**):

1. The functional (and anatomical) lower esophageal sphincter
2. The diaphragmatic hiatus
3. The valvular element of gastric anatomy (angle of His)

> Endoscopy is excellent for evaluating the morphology of this region. A functional evaluation is often subject to a degree of uncertainty and especially to differences of interpretation by different examiners.
>
> The endoscopist identifies and evaluates the sphincter itself, the diaphragmatic hiatus, and the transitional region between the squamous epithelium of the esophagus and the columnar epithelium of the stomach, which are separated by a visible junction called the Z-line.

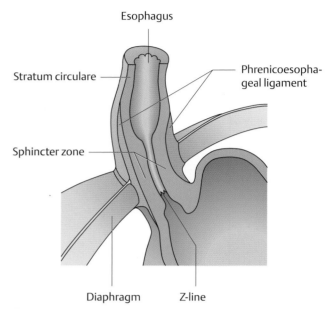

Fig. 2.**20** **Sphincter zone of the terminal esophagus**

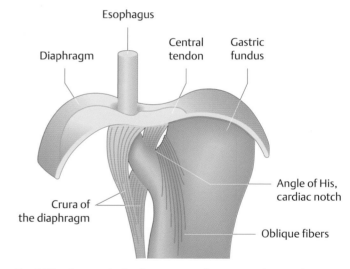

Fig. 2.**21 Anatomical closure mechanisms** about the gastroesophageal junction. The stomach has been slightly separated from the diaphragm for clarity

Lower Esophageal Sphincter and Diaphragmatic Hiatus

■ Anatomy

The lower esophageal sphincter is an approximately 3-cm-long (2–4 cm) segment in the distal esophagus. It can be identified manometrically by its resting pressure of 15–25 mmHg and, less confidently, by its anatomical features. The sphincter zone lies partly above and partly below the diaphragm in the region of the esophageal hiatus. The Z-line in its lower portion marks the boundary between the esophageal squamous epithelium and gastric columnar epithelium (the squamocolumnar junction).

> Endoscopically, the action of the tightly closed sphincter in a healthy subject creates a rosette pattern with four to six longitudinal folds in the distal esophagus (Fig. 2.**22 a**). Viewing from a level just above the sphincter, especially with air insufflation, will reveal per-istaltic waves followed by a transient opening of the sphincter segment, briefly exposing the Z-line and the interior of the stomach (Fig. 2.**22 b, c**). Following careful inspection of this region, the endoscope is gently advanced at a moment when the sphincter is relaxed. The action of the diaphragm muscles can often be seen as respiration-dependent luminal constrictions, especially if the sphincter does not close too tightly. The examiner evaluates the sphincter segment, its distance from the incisor teeth, its functional competence, and the diaphragmatic hiatus. It is particularly important to assess whether the lower esophageal sphincter is competent or incompetent, although this assessment varies considerably among different examiners. The position of the diaphragmatic hiatus is also assessed in relation to the incisor teeth, the lower esophageal sphincter, and the Z-line.

Fig. 2.**22 Passage through the gastroesophageal junction**

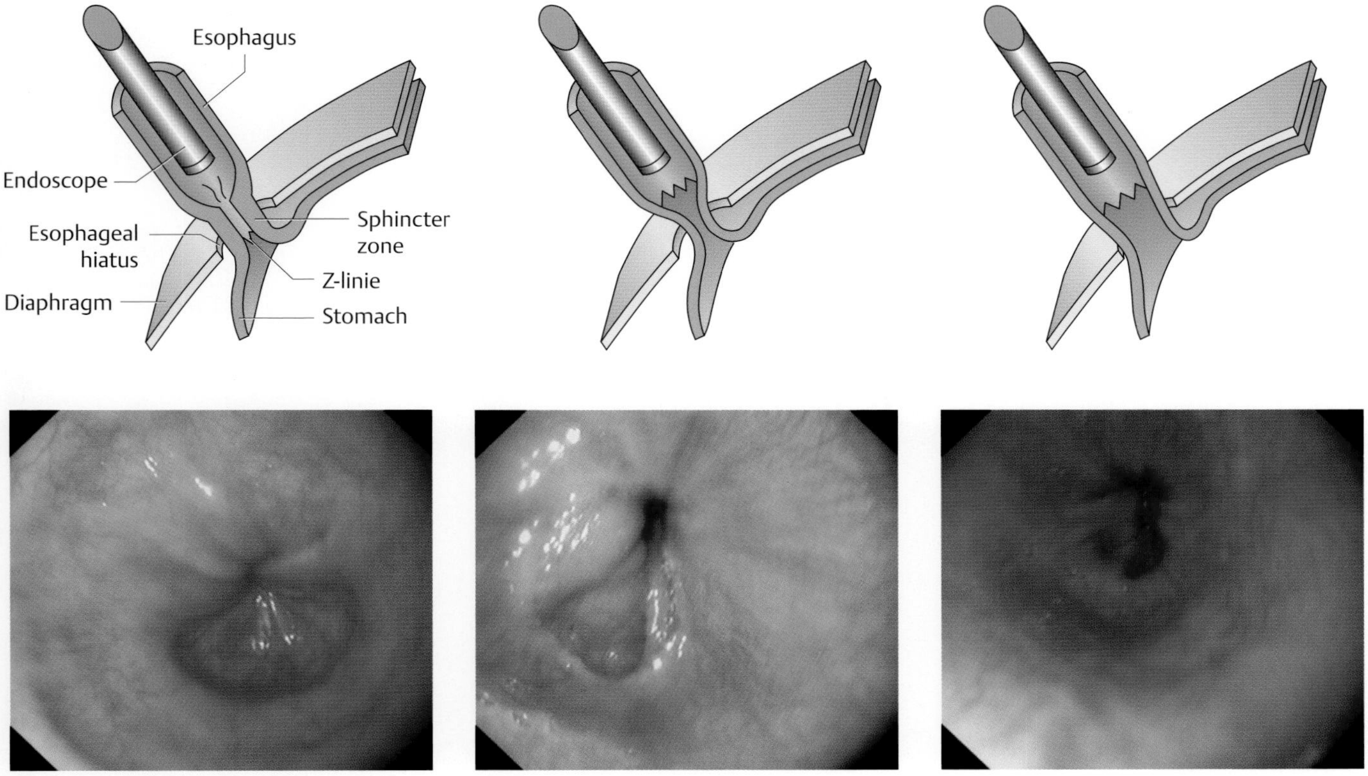

a The sphincter is closed and shows a typical rosettelike appearance

b The sphincter is starting to open, exposing the Z-line in the lower part of the sphincter region

c The sphincter is open, exposing the interior of the stomach. The areas proximal and distal to the Z-line can now be clearly evaluated

Z-Line

■ Anatomy

The Z-line, the boundary between the esophageal and gastric epithelium, should be identified, localized, and evaluated in every upper endoscopy. The location of the Z-line is measured in centimeters from the incisor teeth, with a normal range of 36–40 cm. The relation of the line to the esophageal hiatus should also be described. This relation is variable and depends upon respiration, the axial pressure applied with the endoscope, and constitutional factors. The Z-line is located at or slightly above the level of the esophageal hiatus.

The endoscopic appearance of the Z-line is highly variable (Fig. 2.**23**). It usually has a jagged or undulating shape and is basically symmetrical. The gastric mucosa appears redder, fresher, and slightly raised in relation to the pale pink or gray epithelium of the esophagus. The boundary line may be very irregular; "flames" of gastric mucosa may project into the esophagus, just as tongues of esophageal epithelium may extend downward. These extensions may be largely uniform and symmetrical, or they may have a completely asymmetrical aspect. Occasionally the epithelial boundary appears blurred or indistinct, but usually it is sharply defined. The line may show hypertrophic thickening or may even form a functionally active ring.

Fig. 2.**23 Shape of the Z-line**

Schematic diagrams and illustrative endoscopic images.
The normal range of variation is large.

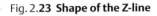

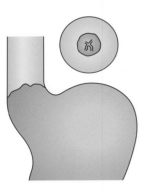 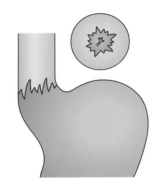 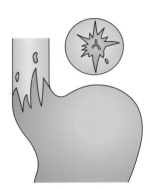

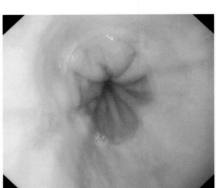 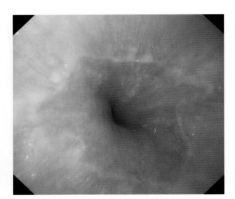 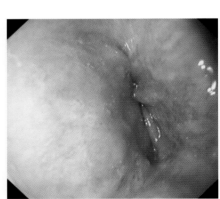

a Ring-shaped   **b** Jagged   **c** Flame-shaped

Swallowing and Esophageal Motility

Endoscopy is not the best method for evaluating esophageal motility and its disorders. Nor is it useful for characterizing esophageal motility due to artifacts caused by air insufflation, stretching of the esophageal wall, contact with the endoscope, and gagging by the patient. Nevertheless, relatively gross abnormalities of esophageal motility can be appreciated during endoscopy. The examiner should take time to observe esophageal peristalsis, particularly when investigating swallowing difficulties, obstruction-related symptoms, and noncardiac chest pain.

■ Physiology

Spontaneous peristaltic activity is not present in the normal esophagus. Swallowing triggers an orderly sequence of muscular relaxation alternating with waves of peristaltic contraction. In the approximately 3-cm-long zone of the upper esophageal sphincter, swallowing initially causes the intraluminal pressure to fall from approximately 80 mmHg to zero, followed by a powerful contraction. This process is transmitted down the esophagus reflexly and by peristalsis: contraction of the circular muscles above the food bolus and relaxation of the muscles below the bolus, with concomitant shortening of the esophagus by contraction of the longitudinal muscles. The initiation of swallowing rapidly induces a drop in pressure at the lower esophageal sphincter, well before the contraction wave reaches the lower esophagus (Fig. 2.**24**).

This complex process, called primary peristalsis, is observed only partially during endoscopy. It is accompanied by orderly contractions of the circular muscles induced by the endoscope itself (secondary peristalsis) and by broad, simultaneous, nonpropulsive contractions that occur at various levels of the esophagus (tertiary

peristalsis). Gagging is associated with fine contractions that cause a rippling of the esophageal surface. Bizarre patterns are occasionally caused by contractions of the circular and longitudinal muscles. These phenomena of esophageal motility are observed even in healthy, asymptomatic patients. Abnormalities of esophageal motility like those seen in achalasia (p. 81 f.) and nutcracker esophagus are described in a later section (p. 84 f.).

■ Terminology of Esophageal Motility

Primary Peristalsis

Primary peristalsis refers to the propulsive waves of contraction that are evoked by normal swallowing and travel down the entire esophagus. They can be observed during endoscopy when the patient swallows.

Secondary Peristalsis

This refers to propulsive contractions that are triggered by local stimuli within the esophagus and are transmitted by normal peristaltic activity. They may be initiated by a large food bolus, reflux, or by endoscopy. Physiologically, secondary peristalsis is one of the clearance mechanisms of the esophagus. Absence of this activity may signify a motility disorder (achalasia, scleroderma).

Tertiary Peristalsis

This refers to nonpropulsive, irregular contractions that may occur synchronously in some circumstances. They may be observed during endoscopy in a healthy subject, and their physiological function is unknown.

Fig. 2.**24 Esophageal peristalsis**

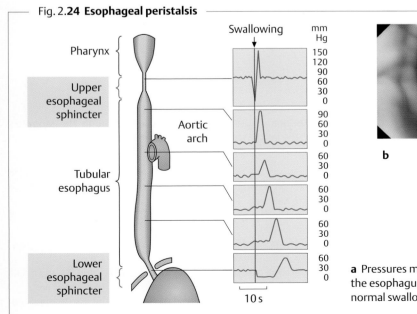

a Pressures measured in the esophagus during normal swallowing

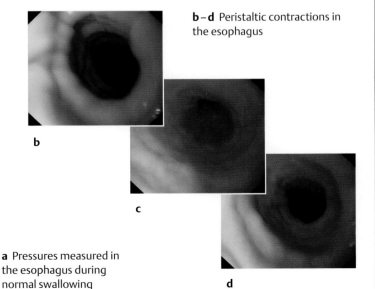

b–d Peristaltic contractions in the esophagus

Examining the Stomach During Insertion

■ Technical Aspects

After the instrument has passed through the esophageal hiatus, the interior of the stomach can be viewed. The various regions of the stomach are evaluated during instrument insertion and withdrawal. The exact sequence of the systematic examination depends on the endoscopist. Here we shall cover the technical aspects of surveying the stomach during insertion and then describe how specific regions of the stomach are evaluated.

 The first region that is seen after entry is the junction of the fundus and body of the stomach. Usually there is a small pool of resting juice, which should be carefully removed by suction to minimize the risk of reflux and aspiration and to aid subsequent inspection of the fundus (Fig. 2.**25**).

■ Advancing the Endoscope

A clear luminal view is often difficult to obtain initially, particularly if the patient cannot retain the insufflated air. It is helpful, therefore, to mentally picture the course of the gastric lumen and the endoscope maneuvers that will have to be performed (Fig. 2.**26**).

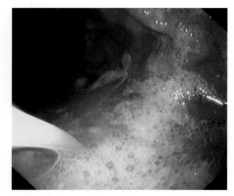

Fig. 2.25 Entering the stomach
a Pool of fluid on the greater curvature. Typical view upon entering the stomach (left side of image: string of mucus)

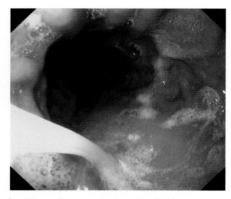

b View after suctioning the fluid

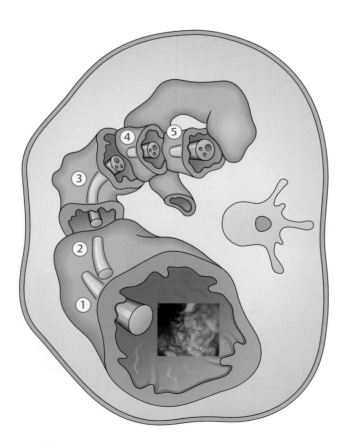

Fig. 2.26 Route of the endoscope passage through the stomach. Notice that the initial view depends on the rotational position of the endoscope

1. Advancing toward the gastric body. The instrument tip is angled slightly forward and toward the lesser curve, and the shaft is rotated slightly to the left.
2. The endoscope is straightened, advanced, and rotated slightly to the right (clockwise).
3. The endoscope is advanced with the tip angled slightly upward, passing below the ridgelike angulus.
4. The endoscope is advanced, straightened, and rotated slightly to the right.
5. The pylorus is centered in the field of view, and the endoscope is advanced toward it.

Views: Fundus–Body Junction and Gastric Body

Fig. 2.**27 View of the fundus–body junction**

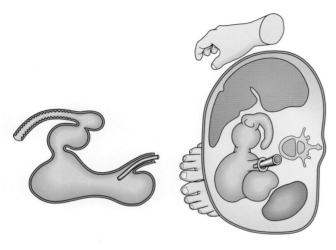
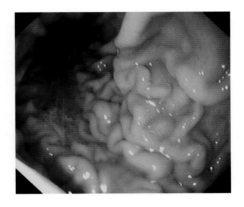

View 1

The endoscope tip is straight upon entering the stomach. The gastric body is visible at the 9-o'clock position in the distant part of the field. The initial part of the fluid pool that is usually seen in the fundus is visible at the 3-o'clock position. The lesser curvature is in the 12-o'clock position, and the greater curvature is at the 6-o'clock position. As the endoscope is advanced further and air is added, the instrument tip usually must be rotated slightly to the left and simultaneously raised by turning the inner wheel toward the endoscopist. This maneuver directs the endoscope tip toward the lesser curvature, and rotating the shaft to the left directs the scope anteriorly where most of the gastric body is located. At this stage the tip has reached the central portion of the gastric body (view 2).

Fig. 2.**28 Midbody region of the stomach**

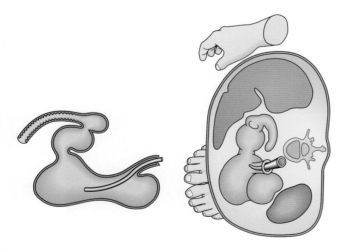
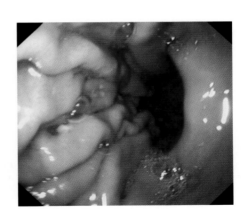

View 2

This view displays the more or less constricted lumen of the gastric body, which exhibits a prominent pattern of mucosal folds. The lumen curves out of view in the background. This view is similar to looking into a horn: You look from the base of the horn toward the tip, which is located at the end of a gentle sweep at upper right and cannot be seen. Vision is often less than optimal at this stage because the gastric body is mostly deflated, but the luminal view should be adequate for further insertion. The endoscope is now straightened somewhat, advanced along the luminal axis, and rotated slightly to the right (clockwise), and the instrument tip is angled slightly upward again. With adequate air insufflation, the junction of the gastric body and antrum comes into view as the endoscope is advanced further (view 3).

Views: Body–Antrum Junction and Antrum

Fig. 2.**29 View into the body–antrum junction**

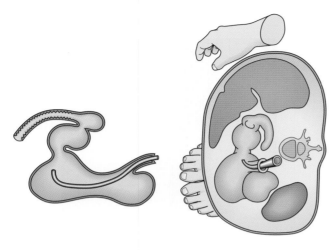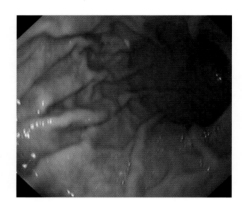

View 3

The hornlike shape of the body–antrum junctional region is clearly appreciated in this view. The ridge of the angulus on the lesser curvature, located at the 12-o'clock position, restricts vision into the more distant antrum. Opposite the angulus, at the 6-o'clock position, are the diminishing rugal folds of the gastric body. The anterior wall of the stomach is at the 9-o'clock position, the posterior wall is at the 3-o'clock position. The instrument is slowly advanced with the tip raised, not rotating the shaft, until the tip passes beneath the angulus and into the antrum (view 4).

Fig. 2.**30 View into the antrum**

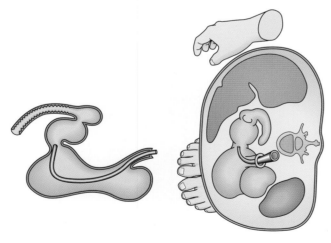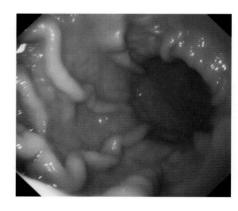

View 4

The instrument is now at the center of the antrum. Peristaltic waves sweep past the instrument tip, traveling down the antrum toward the pylorus. The presence of these waves, which are highly variable in their frequency, constantly alters the appearance of the antrum. The endoscope is advanced slowly. The pylorus is visualized by rotating the endoscope slightly to the right, which advances the tip posteriorly. Now the tip is advanced slowly toward the pylorus, accompanied by a slight straightening maneuver. The pylorus is centered in the image (view 5).

Views: Pylorus

Fig. 2.**31 View of the pylorus**

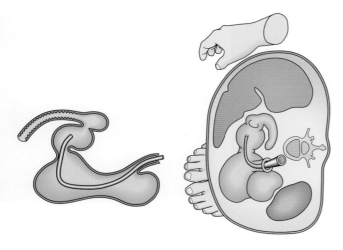 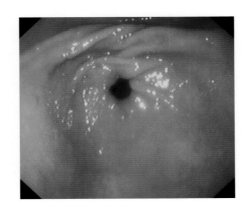

View 5

The pylorus usually appears as a small orifice whose appearance is constantly changing due to antral peristalsis. The size of the opening is variable, ranging from punctate to gaping. The endoscope is advanced slowly, timing the advance to coincide with peristaltic waves. At this time the endoscope may form a redundant loop along the greater curvature and antrum. Thus, as the endoscope is pushed forward, the shaft bows into the antrum without advancing the instrument tip (see p. 42).

At this point the tip of the endoscope should be stationed directly in front of the pylorus (view 6).

Fig. 2.**32 Views: Pylorus**

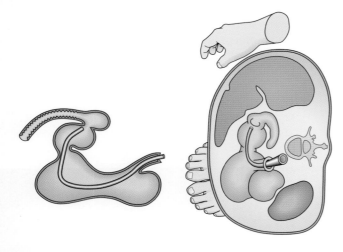 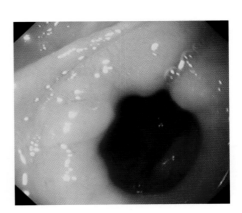

View 6

In this view the pylorus has opened following a peristaltic wave. Intubating the pylorus is usually difficult for the novice, who should try to center the orifice and keep withdrawing and advancing the instrument. The help of an experienced assistant who knows just when to advance the instrument is critical in this situation. After passing through the pylorus, the endoscope tip is in the duodenal bulb (Fig. 2.**39**).

Gastric Body

■ Details

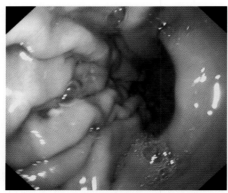 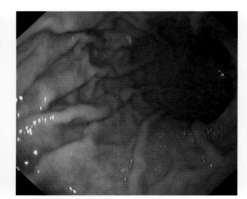 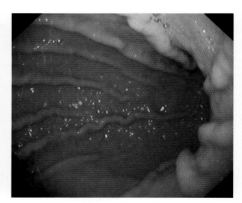

Fig. 2.**33** **Variable shape of the gastric body.** The shape of the body lumen depends on its degree of distension by air insufflation
a Slightly distended

b Moderately distended

c Strongly distended

 The following details should be observed and evaluated in the gastric body.

▶ **Shape**
The body appears as a funnel-shaped cavity that tapers down to a constriction at the angulus. Before air is insufflated, it is in a collapsed state (Fig. 2.33).

▶ **Surface**
Inspection in the collapsed state shows a seemingly random pattern of tortuous mucosal folds on the greater curvature side. When air is added, the folds straighten out and may be effaced when the lumen is maximally distended. Smaller folds run along the lesser curvature and along the anterior and posterior walls into the deeper part of the stomach (Fig. 2.**34**).

▶ **Topography**
When the endoscope is normally positioned in the gastric body (Fig. 2.**26**), the lesser curvature is located approximately between the 9- and the 12-o'clock positions, opposite the greater curvature. The anterior wall is on the left, the posterior wall on the right.

▶ **Mucosa**
The gastric mucosa is variable in color, usually appearing reddish–orange. The polygon-shaped areae gastricae are frequently observed. Few if any blood vessels are seen, but networks of vessels may be visible through mucosa that is atrophic.

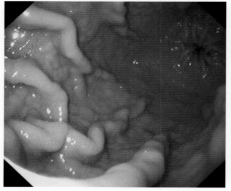 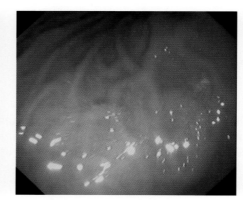 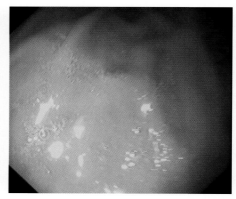

Fig. 2.**34** **Surface structure of the gastric body**
a Distant view. Notice the tortuous rural folds of the gastric body

b Closer view

c Close-up view. The areae gastricae can be seen

Body–Antrum Junction and Antrum

■ Details

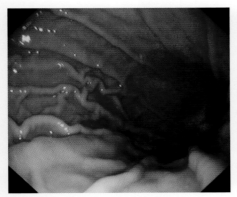

Fig. 2.35 Shape of the body–antrum junction
a Observe the typical tapering of the body toward the antrum

b The angulus marks the transition to the antrum

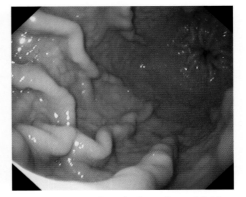

c The antrum is largely free of rugal folds

 The endoscopic details of the body–antrum junction and antrum are reviewed below.

Body–antrum junction

▶ **Shape**
Marked tapering of the stomach is usually noted at the body–antrum junction (Fig. 2.**35**).

▶ **Topography**
The typical curve of the angulus is visible in the distance. It provides a landmark for positively identifying the greater and lesser curves and the anterior and posterior walls.

▶ **Surface**
The gastric folds generally give way to smooth mucosa as you proceed from the body of the stomach to the antrum. In rare cases, folds are seen extending deep into the antrum.

▶ **Mucosa**
The mucosa at the body–antrum junction is reddish–orange, as in the body itself. Often it appears more red, and it may even have a somewhat patchy appearance.

Antrum

▶ **Shape**
The antrum has the shape of a dome with the pylorus at the apex (Figs. 2.**36**–2.**38**).

▶ **Topography**
The greater and lesser curvatures and anterior and posterior walls are easy to identify after you have passed the angulus (Fig. 2.**40**).

▶ **Surface**
The prepyloric folds in the antrum have a highly variable appearance (Fig. 2.**41**).

▶ **Mucosa**
The antral mucosa is smooth and also highly variable in its coloration, which ranges from yellowish–gray to reddish–orange.

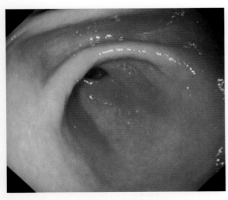

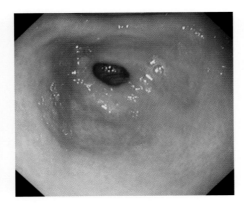

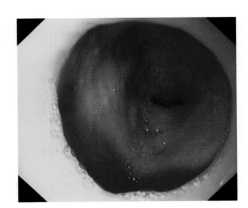

Fig. 2.**36 Advancing toward the pylorus**

Antral Region

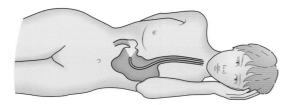

Fig. 2.37 Position of the antrum in left lateral decubitus. The dome of the antrum forms the highest point at which the insufflated air collects

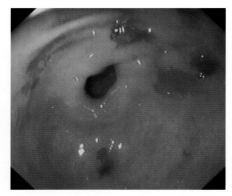

Fig. 2.38 View of the pylorus in the antral dome. Circumferential biopsy samples have been taken. The radial pattern of blood tracks reflects the domelike shape of the antrum

Fig. 2.39 Looping of the endoscope in the stomach

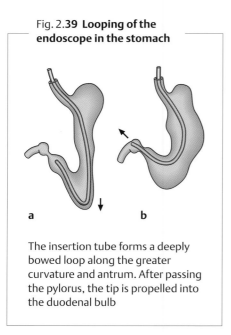

a   b

The insertion tube forms a deeply bowed loop along the greater curvature and antrum. After passing the pylorus, the tip is propelled into the duodenal bulb

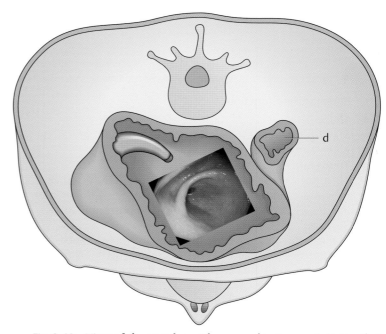

Fig. 2.40 View of the angulus with a curved instrument. Notice that when the angulus region is sharply angled, the inlet and outlet of the stomach are oriented approximately in the same direction
d = duodenum

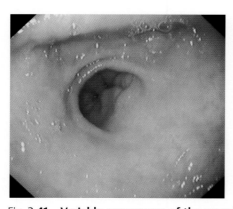
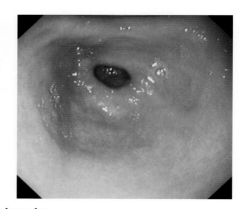
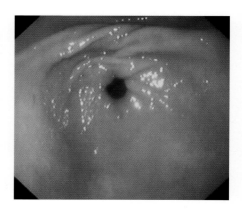

Fig. 2.41 Variable appearance of the prepyloric region

Antral Peristalsis

Fig. 2.**42 Peristaltic waves**

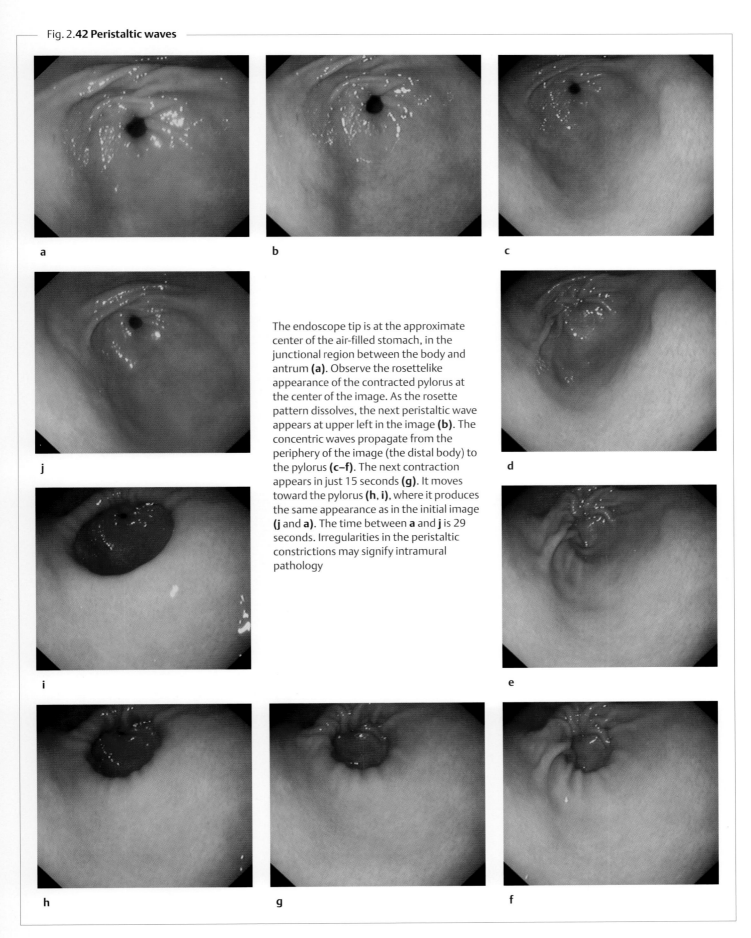

The endoscope tip is at the approximate center of the air-filled stomach, in the junctional region between the body and antrum **(a)**. Observe the rosettelike appearance of the contracted pylorus at the center of the image. As the rosette pattern dissolves, the next peristaltic wave appears at upper left in the image **(b)**. The concentric waves propagate from the periphery of the image (the distal body) to the pylorus **(c–f)**. The next contraction appears in just 15 seconds **(g)**. It moves toward the pylorus **(h, i)**, where it produces the same appearance as in the initial image **(j** and **a)**. The time between **a** and **j** is 29 seconds. Irregularities in the peristaltic constrictions may signify intramural pathology

Retroflexion Maneuver

■ Components of Retroflexion

Since the entire upper gastrointestinal tract is inspected and evaluated with a forward-viewing endoscope, retroflexion is necessary to obtain a complete view of the cardia and fundus. The angulus and body are also examined in retroflexion (Figs. 2.**43**, 2.**44**). The retroflexion maneuver consists of the following components:

▶ The large inner control wheel moves the instrument tip in the plane of the wheel
  – Turning the wheel backward (counterclockwise) deflects the endoscope tip forward and upward into a U shape.
  – Turning the wheel forward (clockwise) deflects the tip backward into a J shape.
▶ The small outer control wheel angles the endoscope tip laterally from the plane of the wheel
  – Turning the wheel backward deflects the tip to the left.
  – Turning the wheel forward deflects the tip to the right.

In the retroflexion maneuver, the instrument tip is deflected upward into a U shape and simultaneously rotated to the right by turning the large wheel backward and the small wheel forward.

Fig. 2.**43** **Retroflexion across the angulus**

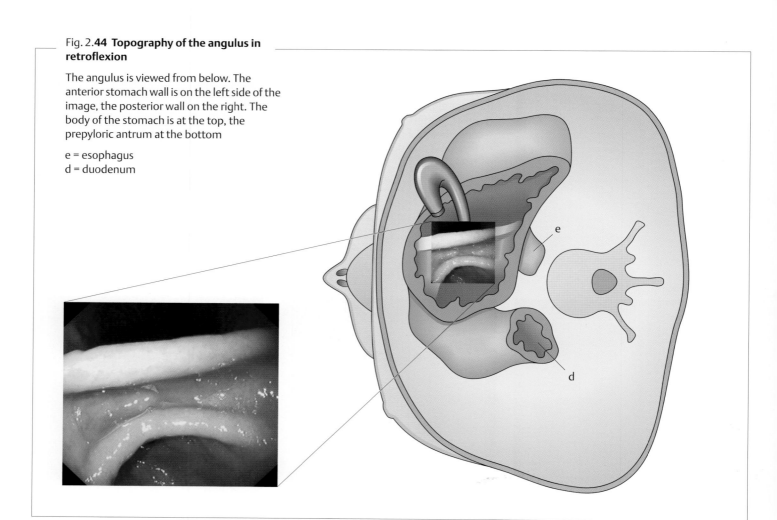

a   b   c

a First the endoscope tip is deflected upward into a U shape
b The endoscope is simultaneously withdrawn and rotated toward the greater curvature
c A combination of angling and twisting movements are used to inspect the cardia and fundus

Fig. 2.**44** **Topography of the angulus in retroflexion**

The angulus is viewed from below. The anterior stomach wall is on the left side of the image, the posterior wall on the right. The body of the stomach is at the top, the prepyloric antrum at the bottom

e = esophagus
d = duodenum

Retroflexion in the Stomach

■ Maneuvering the Endoscope

For retroflexion in the antrum, the instrument tip is angled upward (see p. 44), and the field of view is slowly tracked across the angulus.

The angulus is inspected, and the instrument is slowly withdrawn into the air-distended body of the stomach to inspect the fundus and cardia from below (Fig. 2.**45**).

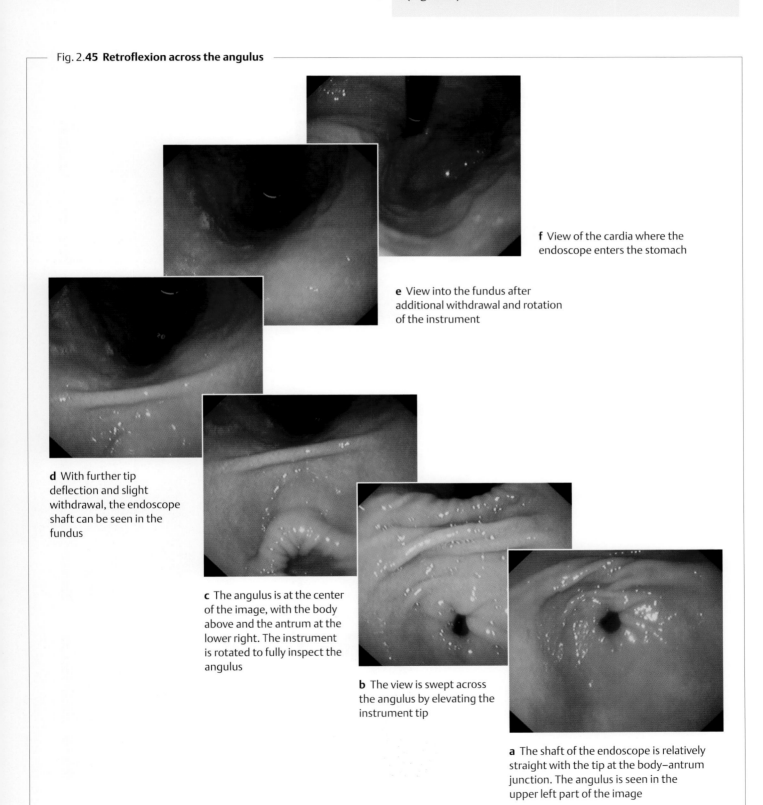

Fig. 2.**45 Retroflexion across the angulus**

f View of the cardia where the endoscope enters the stomach

e View into the fundus after additional withdrawal and rotation of the instrument

d With further tip deflection and slight withdrawal, the endoscope shaft can be seen in the fundus

c The angulus is at the center of the image, with the body above and the antrum at the lower right. The instrument is rotated to fully inspect the angulus

b The view is swept across the angulus by elevating the instrument tip

a The shaft of the endoscope is relatively straight with the tip at the body–antrum junction. The angulus is seen in the upper left part of the image

Inspection of the Fundus

■ Maneuvering the Endoscope

The dome of the fundus is inspected by angling the tip upward and withdrawing the instrument.

Often a small pool of gastric juice can be seen at this location (between the 7- and 9-o'clock positions in Fig. 2.**46a**). The instrument tip can be partially immersed in the pool with the lens protruding (like crocodile eyes) in order to aspirate this fluid. Angling movements are combined with slight rotation to inspect all areas of the fundus (Fig. 2.**46**).

Fig. 2.**46 Gastric fundus**

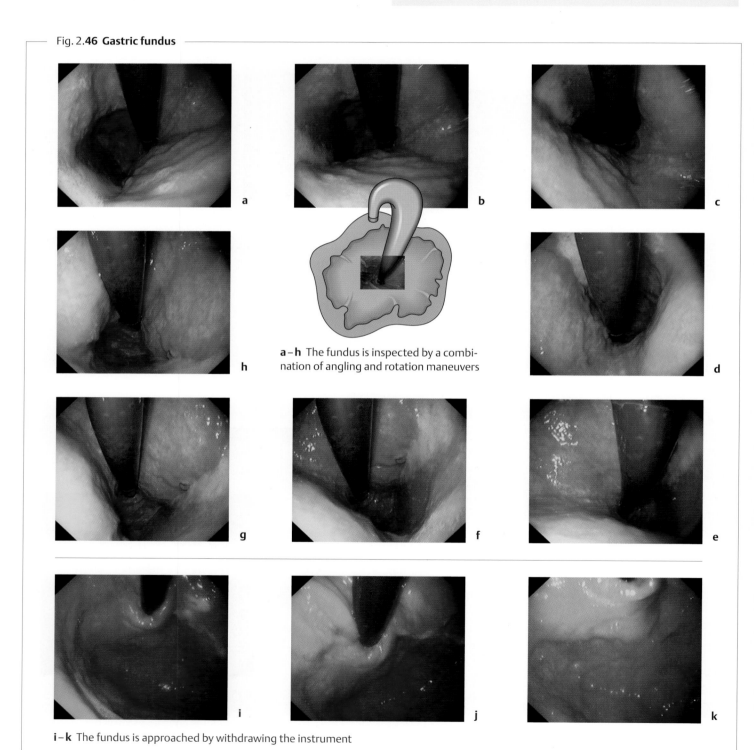

a–h The fundus is inspected by a combination of angling and rotation maneuvers

i–k The fundus is approached by withdrawing the instrument

Inspection of the Cardia

■ Maneuvering the Endoscope

Inspection of the cardia is difficult because the more proximal part of the endoscope shaft partially obscures the cardial region.

Typically the shaft can be seen in the upper part of the retroflexed image. This view demonstrates the prominent fold of the cardiac notch and the dome of the fundus beyond. Frequently the Z-line can be identified, and it is not unusual to see a small epiphrenic ampulla or hiatal hernia. Center the cardia in the image, then rotate the endoscope 180° clockwise and back counterclockwise to inspect all portions of the cardia (Fig. 2.**47**).

Fig. 2.**47 Inspection of the cardia**

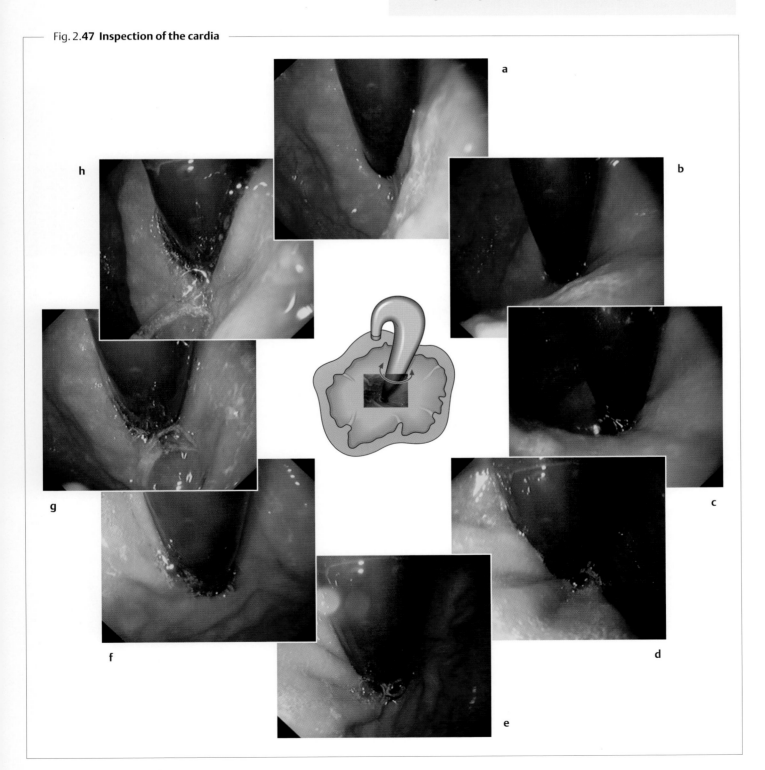

2

Relations of the Stomach: Abdominal Wall

■ Anatomy

The position of the stomach is not constant. It depends on age, body position, and the degree of gastric distension. Organs that are in contact with the stomach can often be identified: the liver, pancreas, heart, and spleen (Table 2.**6**).

■ Identifying the Abdominal Wall

It is important to know the relation of the stomach to the abdominal wall, particularly during the placement of a feeding tube (Figs. 2.**48**–2.**50**).

Table 2.**6**   Relations of the stomach

Anterior wall		Posterior wall	
Cardia **Lesser curvature** **Angulus** **Pylorus**	**Fundus**	**Fundus**	**Body**
Inferior surface of liver	Diaphragm Chest wall Abdominal wall	Spleen Diaphragm Heart	Pancreas Duodenum Spleen

Orientation requires knowing the axis of the endoscope shaft. This forms the basis for identifying the lesser and greater curvatures of the stomach and the anterior and posterior walls (Fig. 2.**51**). The anterior wall can be positively identified by indenting the external abdomen with the finger and looking for the bulge (Fig. 2.**49**).

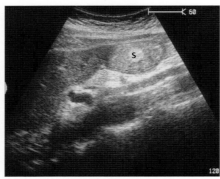
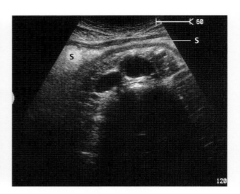

Fig. 2.**50**   **Ultrasound views of the stomach.** The distended stomach is broadly apposed to the abdominal wall
a   Longitudinal scan

b   Transverse scan
    s = stomach

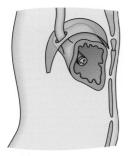

Fig. 2.**48**   **Relation of the stomach to the abdominal wall.** Conventional anatomical view

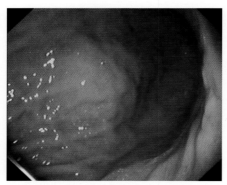

Fig. 2.**49**   **View of the anterior wall of the distended body of the stomach.** The indentation at the 8-o'clock position is caused by digital pressure on the external abdominal wall

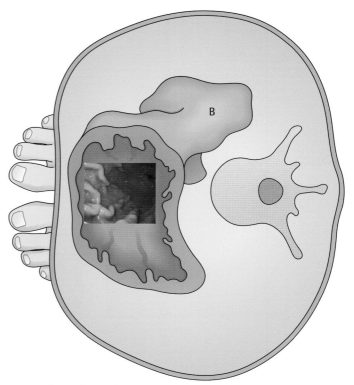

Fig. 2.**51**   **Topography in the endoscopic image.** Straight-ahead view of the stomach and abdominal wall
db = duodenal bulb

Relations of the Stomach: Pancreas

■ Impression from the Pancreas

The pancreas often makes an oblong impression in the area of the body–antrum junction (Figs. 2.**52**–2.**54**). Figure 2.**55** shows the topography in the endoscopic image.

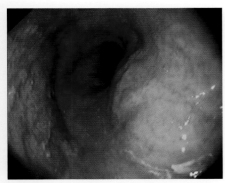

Fig. 2.**52**   **Impression from the pancreas.** Typical appearance of the posterior stomach wall in the area of the body–antrum junction

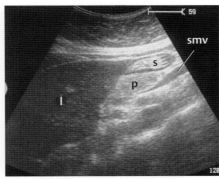

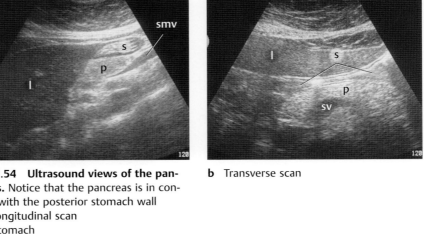

Fig. 2.**54**   **Ultrasound views of the pancreas.** Notice that the pancreas is in contact with the posterior stomach wall
a   Longitudinal scan
s = stomach
p = pancreas
l = liver
sv = splenic vein
smv = superior mesenteric vein

b   Transverse scan

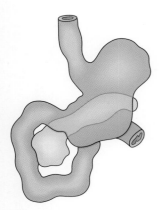

Fig. 2.**53**   **Relation of the stomach and pancreas.** Conventional anatomical view

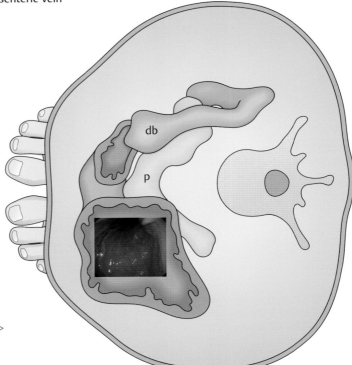

Fig. 2.**55**   **Topography in the endoscopic image.** The location of the ▷ pancreas in the image depends on the rotation of the instrument
db = duodenal bulb
p = pancreas

Relations of the Stomach: Liver

■ Impression from the Inferior Hepatic Border

The inferior border of the liver often appears as a short indentation in the angulus region (Figs. 2.**56**–2.**58**). It is difficult to appreciate the topography in this region due to the looped position of the endoscope in the antrum. The topography is shown in Figure 2.**59**.

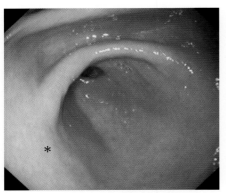

Fig. 2.**56** **Impression from the liver.** Typical appearance of the anterior stomach wall in the angulus region. The impression from the liver is visible between the 7- and 9-o'clock positions (*)

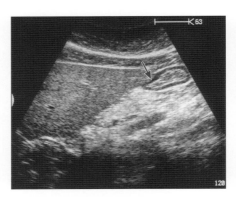
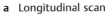
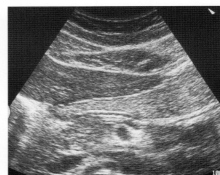

Fig. 2.**58** **Ultrasound views of the hepatic border.** The sharp-angled hepatic border creates a distinct impression in the stomach wall (arrow)
a Longitudinal scan

b Transverse scan

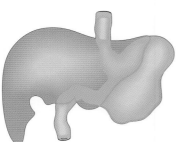
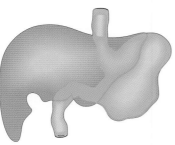

Fig. 2.**57** **Relation of the stomach and liver.** Conventional anatomical view

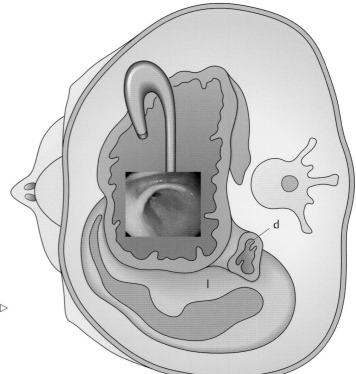

Fig. 2.**59** **Topography in the endoscopic image.** The endoscope is ▷ angled upward in the antrum to view the angulus from below. The liver forms a visible impression in the anterior stomach wall on the left side of the image
l = liver
d = duodenum

Relations of the Stomach: Heart and Spleen

■ Cardiac Notch, Impressions from the Heart and Spleen

The endoscopic appearance of the fundus and cardia is influenced by the adjacent diaphragm, spleen, and and heart. Understanding this appearance requires an adjustment in thinking due to the U-shaped deflection of the endoscope for inspecting the fundus and cardia (Fig. 2.63).

The diaphragm creates the deep fold of the cardiac notch. The impressions from the spleen and heart can be identified in the dome of the fundus (Figs. 2.60–2.63). The spleen may bulge deeply into the fundus, but in some cases it may only flatten the fundus dome and produce a dark discoloration of the gastric mucosa. Distinct cardiac pulsations can usually be seen opposite the splenic impression.

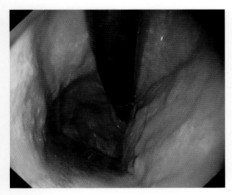

Fig. 2.**60   Normal configuration of the gastric fundus**

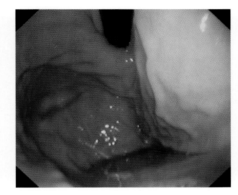

Fig. 2.**61 a, b   Impression from the heart.** Shape changes are seen in the dome of the fundus during cardiac pulsations. The cardiac impression is clearly visible at the center

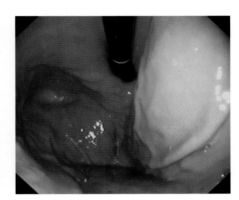

b

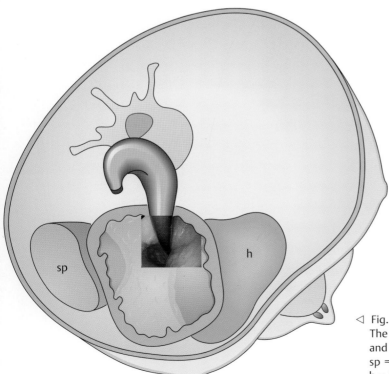

sp

h

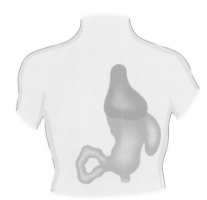

Fig. 2.**62   Relations of the stomach, heart, and spleen.** The heart is in contact with the stomach superiorly and anteriorly; the spleen superiorly, posteriorly, and laterally

◁ Fig. 2.**63   Cross section at the level of the fundus.** Caudocranial view. The retroflexed endoscope is shown. The impressions from the heart and spleen are visible, along with a small pool of fluid
sp = spleen
h = heart

Passage into the Duodenal Bulb

■ Passing the Endoscope

The endoscope tip often passes swiftly into the duodenal bulb due to the looped position of the instrument shaft along the greater curve and antrum. When the pylorus opens in this situation, the endoscope slips quickly into the bulb (Fig. 2.**39**). Usually the bulb is inspected during instrument withdrawal, but often it can be adequately inspected during insertion. In contrast to the stomach, it is difficult to become oriented in the bulbar and proximal duodenum due to the looped position of the endoscope and the various tip deflections that are used.

Usually a small pool of fluid is seen within the duodenal bulb, located between the 11- and 1-o'clock positions in the endoscopic view (Fig. 2.**64**). This fluid collects at the most dependent site in the bulb and thus provides a useful landmark when it is known that the patient is in left lateral decubitus. The true orientation of the organs is shown in Figure 2.**65 a**. The image is displayed upside down due to the looped position of the endoscope. The endoscopist's perspective is shown in Figure 2.**65 b**.

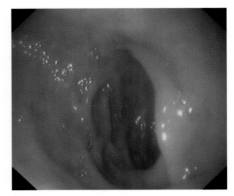

Fig. 2.**64**   **View into the duodenal bulb.** A small pool of fluid is visible at approximately the 11-o'clock position

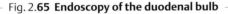
Fig. 2.**65 Endoscopy of the duodenal bulb**

ded = descending duodenum
db = duodenal bulb
e = esophagus
s = stomach

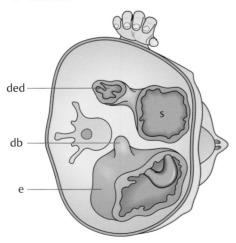

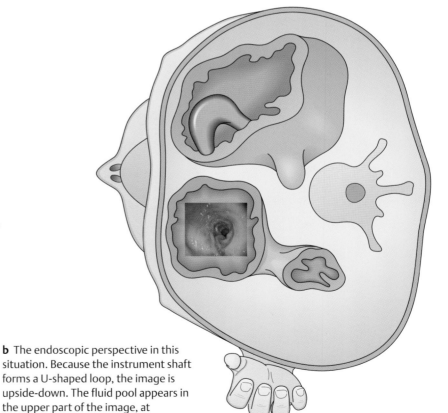

a Anatomy of duodenal bulb endoscopy, viewed from below in true orientation. The patient is lying on the left side. The duodenal bulb lies above the stomach, and some fluid collects at the most dependent site in the bulb

b The endoscopic perspective in this situation. Because the instrument shaft forms a U-shaped loop, the image is upside-down. The fluid pool appears in the upper part of the image, at approximately the 11-o'clock position

Passage into the Descending Duodenum

■ Maneuvering the Endoscope

The novice often has difficulty passing the endoscope from the bulb into the descending duodenum. To understand the necessary maneuvers, note that the endoscope as a whole forms a U-shaped loop and that the flexible tip lies within the bulb in a more or less straightened position. The bulb is located cranial and slightly lateral to the pylorus and extends posteriorly to the junction of the bulbar and descending duodenum at the superior duodenal angle. From there the duodenum descends in the familiar C-shaped arch.

Retroflexing, Rotating, and Advancing the Scope

The endoscope is advanced through the bulb to the superior duodenal angle. From this vantage point, the first valvulae conniventes can be seen. To pass into the descending duodenum, the endoscope is advanced just until it abuts on the distal bulb wall. Now three things must occur simultaneously. The endoscope is:

1. Retroflexed at the tip by turning the control wheels,
2. Rotated clockwise, and
3. Slightly advanced.

This has the following effects: The retroflexion maneuver raises the endoscope tip out of the plane of the diagram (**1** in Fig. 2.**66**). Rotating the shaft to the right (**2**) angles the deflected tip into the introitus of the descending duodenum, and simultaneously advancing the shaft (**3**) moves the endoscope farther down the descending limb.

This maneuver can be reproduced with the hand (Fig. 2.**67**). Hold your left arm in front of you in a supinated position and look at the palm. Now angle the palm toward you (retroflexion) and rotate the forearm to the right (clockwise rotation) while moving the arm forward (advancing). The hand now points into the descending duodenum.

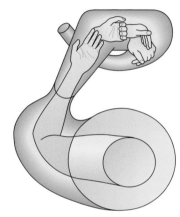

Fig. 2.**67** **Passage through the duodenal bulb.** The left hand demonstrates the spiraling motion around the superior duodenal angle

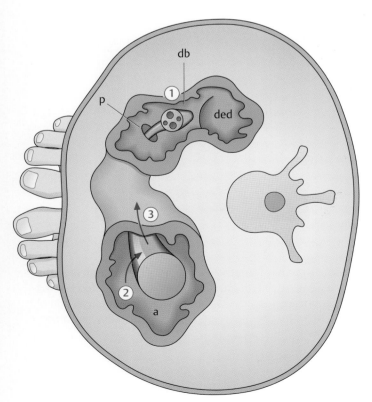

Fig. 2.**66** **Passage into the descending duodenum.** The necessary maneuvers are shown: **1** retroflexing the tip, **2** rotating to the right, **3** advancing
p = pylorus
db = duodenal bulb
ded = descending duodenum
a = antrum

Views: Bulbar and Proximal Duodenum

Fig. 2.**68 Anterior and posterior walls of the duodenal bulb**

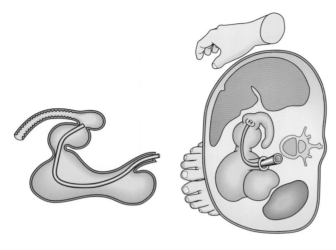 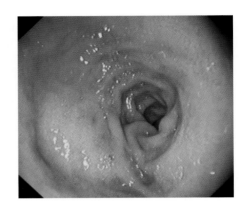

View 7

The instrument tip is in the pylorus. The view is the same, regardless of whether the instrument is advanced or withdrawn: The duodenal bulb appears as a "bulbous" or cylindrical structure of variable length. With a standard instrument position, the junction of the bulb with the second part of the duodenum will be located below and to the right. Try to distinguish between the anterior and posterior walls of the bulb. This is aided by knowing the position of the patient and that the endoscope forms a U-shaped loop in the stomach, turning the image "upside down" (analogous to bending the head far backward and seeing the edge of the upper eyelid at the bottom of the visual field).

Fig. 2.**69 Entrance to the descending duodenum**

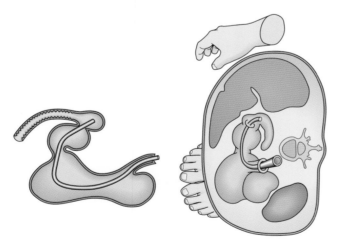 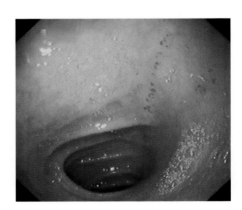

View 8

On reaching the entrance to the descending duodenum, you can see the first valvulae conniventes. The lumen of the duodenum continues downward and to the right from the endoscopist's perspective. The deflection/rotation/advance maneuver for entering the descending duodenum was described above. When this maneuver is completed, the instrument tip should be within the descending duodenum. Evaluation was not possible during insertion of the scope. In the next step, the instrument is slowly withdrawn.

Fig. 2.**70 Descending duodenum**

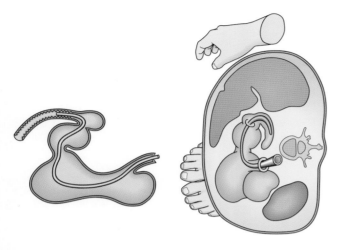

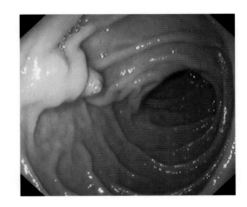

View 9

The complex maneuver described above usually advances the endoscope tip quickly down the descending duodenum. When the instrument is now pulled back, the redundant loop of shaft within the stomach straightens out, causing the endoscope tip to advance again by several centimeters. The lumen is centered in the image, and the duodenum is evaluated while the endoscope is withdrawn. The papillary region is easily recognized but cannot be adequately evaluated with a forward-viewing instrument.

The descending duodenum in view 9 has been distended with air. The valvulae conniventes are clearly visible, and the papilla of Vater can be seen at the 10-o'clock position. Further withdrawal should be done carefully, as the endoscope can easily slip out of the duodenum and fall back into the stomach.

Fig. 2.**71 Junction of the bulbar and descending duodenum**

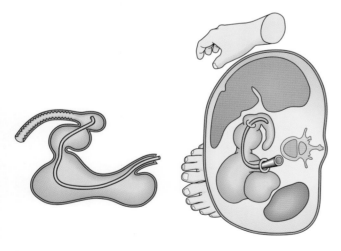

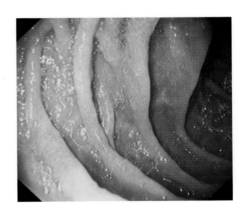

View 10

View 10 shows the typical appearance of the junction of the bulbar and descending duodenum. With the instrument straightened, the view is directed almost at right angles toward the duodenal wall. This view is proximal to view 9 anatomically, but comes after it in the examination sequence. Additional withdrawal will return to the position at view 8.

Inspection of the duodenal bulb requires patience and "feel." The endoscope tip is very unstable when just distal to the pylorus and can easily fall back into the antrum. Lesions in the posterior wall of the bulb are easily missed in this situation, since the straightened endoscope tip extending through the pylorus is aimed at the anterior wall of the bulb.

Duodenal Bulb

■ Details

 The following structural details are noted during endoscopy:

▶ **Shape**
  – With air insufflation: rounded, bulbous, occasionally oblong (Fig. 2.**72**)

▶ **Topography in the endoscopic image** (Fig. 2.**76**)
  – Above: lesser curvature
  – Below: greater curvature

  – Right: posterior wall
  – Left: anterior wall

▶ **Surface** (Figs. 2.**73**, 2.**74**)
  – With air insufflation: almost without folds
  – Distant view: relatively smooth
  – Color: yellowish–gray
  – Frequent: contact bleeding from the instrument tip on the anterior bulb wall (Fig. 2.**75**)

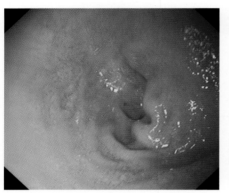

Fig. 2.**72** **Normal duodenal bulb.** Notice the rounded, oblong shape

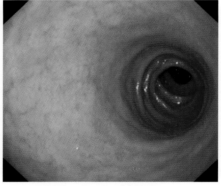

Fig. 2.**73** **Normal duodenal bulb.** Notice the granular mucosal surface

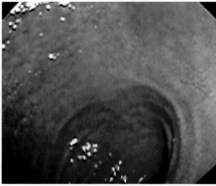

Fig. 2.**74** **Normal duodenal bulb.** The relatively coarse granular pattern of the mucosa is a normal variant

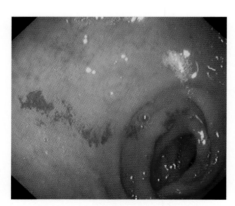

Fig. 2.**75** **Typical contact bleeding.** This occurred when the instrument tip was initially propelled into the duodenal bulb. It is generally located on the anterior wall of the bulb

s = stomach
p = pancreas
a = aorta
d = duodenum
l = liver
ga = gastroduodenal artery
ha = hepatic artery

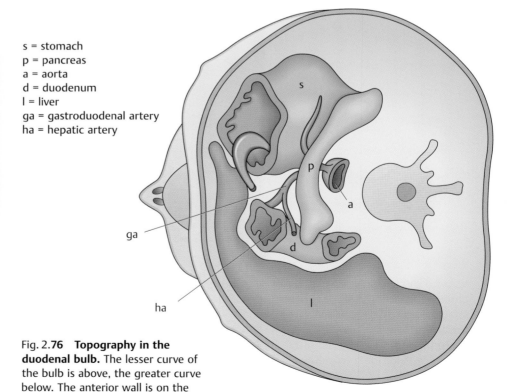

Fig. 2.**76** **Topography in the duodenal bulb.** The lesser curve of the bulb is above, the greater curve below. The anterior wall is on the left, the posterior wall on the right

Descending Duodenum

■ Details

 The details of the descending duodenum are as follows:

▶ **Shape** (Fig. 2.**77**)
  – Curved tunnel
  – Typical: valvulae conniventes
▶ **Topography**
  – Difficult to appreciate spatial orientation
  – Aid orientation by identifying the Vater papilla at approximately the 9-o'clock position (Fig. 2.**80**)
▶ **Surface**
  – Valvulae conniventes
  – Finely granular mucosal pattern (Figs. 2.**78**, 2.**79**)

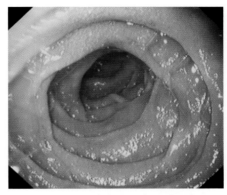

Fig. 2.**77** **Normal descending duodenum**

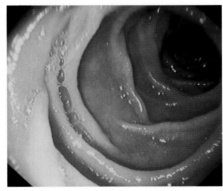

Fig. 2.**78** **Normal descending duodenum.** Notice the fine granularity of the mucosal surface

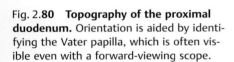

Fig. 2.**80** **Topography of the proximal duodenum.** Orientation is aided by identifying the Vater papilla, which is often visible even with a forward-viewing scope.

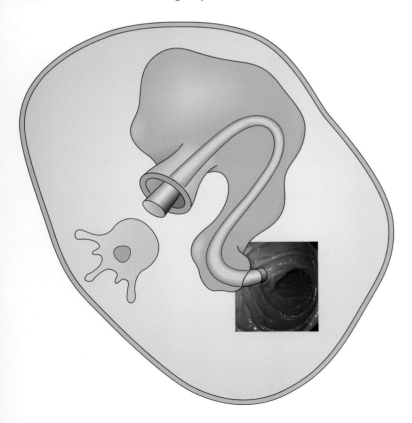

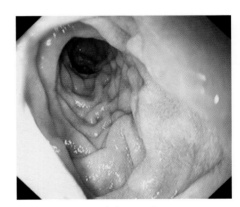

Fig. 2.**79** **Normal descending duodenum.** Relatively coarse granular pattern of the mucosa

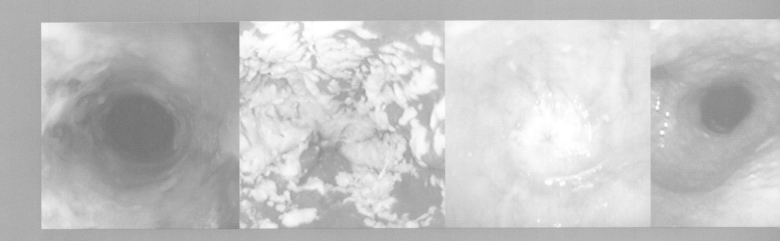

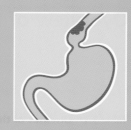
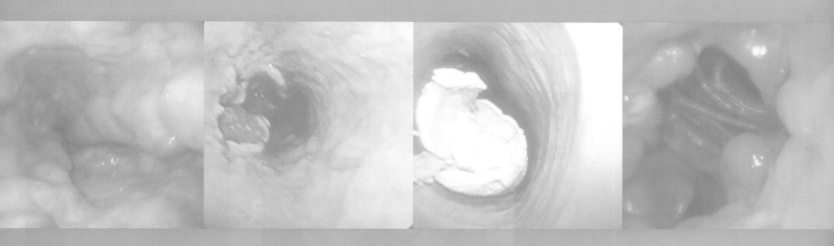

Hiatal Hernia: Axial Sliding Hernia

■ Definitions and Clinical Aspects

Hiatal hernia is defined as the persistent or recurrent herniation of portions of the stomach through the esophageal hiatus into the chest cavity.

An axial sliding hernia is among the most common endoscopic findings, noted in up to 25% of upper gastrointestinal examinations (Fig. 3.**11**). In 80% of cases it is an incidental finding that is classified as a normal variant. The significance of a sliding hernia in the pathogenesis of reflux disease is uncertain. While more than 80% of cases are asymptomatic and endoscopy shows no signs of reflux esophagitis, a sliding hernia is commonly found in cases where esophagitis is already present.

■ Diagnosis

 Endoscopic diagnostic criteria

▶ Forward view (Fig. 3.**11 a, c**)
- Double-ring configuration with an intervening, bell-shaped dilatation. The proximal ring is formed by the lower esophageal sphincter (LES), the distal ring by the esophageal hiatus.
- The gastroesophageal boundary (Z-line) is within the dilated segment, several centimeters above the esophageal hiatus.
- Shortened distance between the Z-line and incisor teeth
- Radial folds passing into the hiatus in the lower part of the hernia
▶ Retroflexed view (Fig. 3.**11 b, c**)
- Cardia does not close snugly around the endoscope
- Bell-shaped dilatation over the cardia
- Folds radiating into the hernia
- Ascent of the hernia during inspiration
▶ **Caution:** Do not pull the retroflexed tip into the esophagus. If this occurs, push back and then straighten the endoscope.

Differential diagnosis

▶ The typical appearance is unmistakable.
▶ Small hernias are often classified as a normal variant.

Checklist for endoscopic evaluation

▶ Distance of the Z-line from the incisor teeth in centimeters
▶ If determinable: distance of the LES from the incisor teeth in centimeters
▶ Distance of the esophageal hiatus from the incisor teeth
▶ Retroflexed view showing lack of cardial closure around the endoscope
▶ Evidence of reflux disease

Additional Study

▶ Oral contrast examination with a head-down tilt (only half of radiographically detectable sliding hernias are visible endoscopically)

Comments

Axial sliding hernia is a common finding and is frequently asymptomatic. With symptomatic reflux, initial treatment consists of supportive measures and proton pump inhibitors (PPI). If medical therapy is unsuccessful or if gastric contents are regurgitated, fundoplication should be performed.

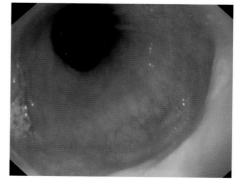

Fig. 3.**11   Axial sliding hernia**
a   Forward view

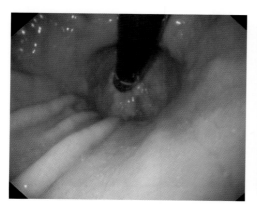

b   Retroflexed view

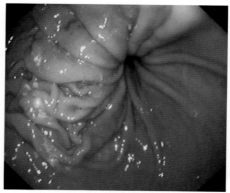

c   Very large hernia in forward view

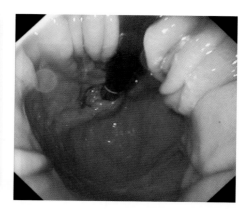

d   Very large hernia in retroflexed view

Hiatal Hernia: Paraesophageal Hernia

■ Definition

Paraesophageal hernia is rare, accounting for less than 5% of all hernias (Fig. 3.**13**). In this condition, portions of the gastric fundus are herniated into the mediastinum. This usually occurs on the greater curvature side, owing to the relatively firm attachment of the lesser curvature to the cardia. Because the lower esophageal sphincter and cardia are normally positioned, this type of hernia can be seen only with a retroflexed endoscope.

■ Diagnosis

 Endoscopic diagnostic criteria

▶ Visible only in retroflexion (Fig. 3.**12**)
▶ Normal configuration of the cardia
▶ Next to the normal cardia is a second lumen, with mucosal folds radiating into it
▶ **Caution:** Avoid entering the hernia with the retroflexed scope.

Differential diagnosis

▶ The typical appearance is unmistakable.

Checklist for endoscopic evaluation

▶ Inspect the hernia in retroflexion.
▶ Check for associated axial sliding hernia (common).
▶ Complications?
▶ Ulceration, necrosis, and incarceration are rarely detectable by endoscopy.

Additional Study

▶ Radiographic contrast examination

Comments

As there is a potential for incarceration, surgical correction is recommended even for asymptomatic cases (gastropexy, fundoplication for combined hernias).

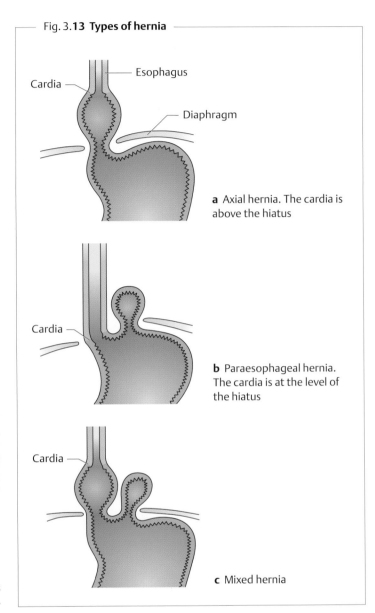

Fig. 3.**13 Types of hernia**

a Axial hernia. The cardia is above the hiatus

b Paraesophageal hernia. The cardia is at the level of the hiatus

c Mixed hernia

3

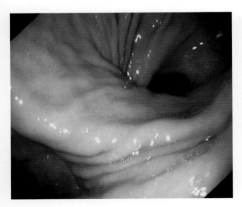

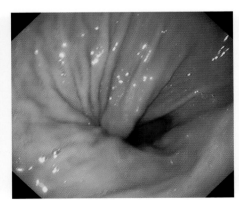

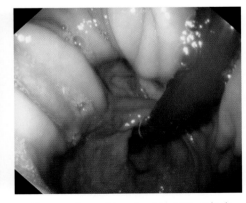

Fig. 3.**12 Paraesophageal hernias**
a Retroflexed view demonstrates the hernia at the 2-o'clock position

b Close-up view

c Paraesophageal hernia at the 12-o'clock position

Hiatal Hernia: Upside-Down Stomach

■ Definition

Upside-down stomach is an extreme form of paraesophageal hernia in which the entire stomach has herniated and rotated upward through the diaphragm into the mediastinum (Fig. 3.**14**).

■ Diagnosis

 Endoscopic diagnostic criteria

▶ Bizarre presentation (Fig. 3.**15**)
▶ Difficult orientation
▶ It is difficult or impossible to reach the pylorus.

Differential diagnosis

▶ None

Checklist for endoscopic evaluation

▶ Inflammatory signs in the esophagus
▶ Inflammatory signs in the stomach

Additional Studies

▶ Plain chest radiograph (Fig. 3.**16**)
▶ Radiographic contrast examination

Comments

The diagnosis is established by contrast radiographs. Surgical correction is advised for patients who are well enough to tolerate surgery.

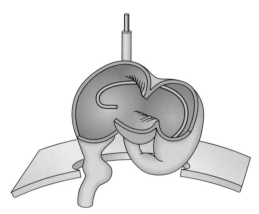

Fig. 3.**14** **Schematic diagram of upside-down stomach.** Complete herniation of the stomach into the chest

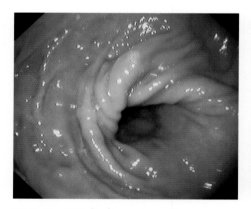
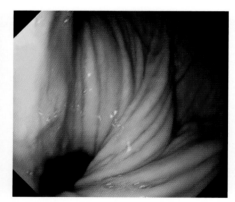
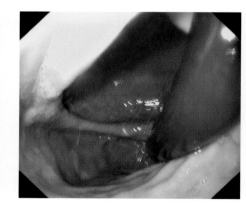

Fig. 3.**15** **Upside-down stomach**
a Herniation through the diaphragm

b Appearance of the cardia region

c Fundus

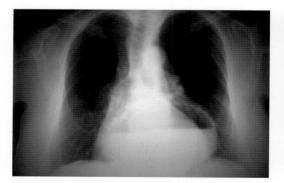
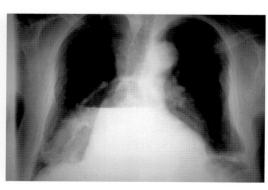

Fig. 3.**16** **Radiographic findings**
a Very large hiatal hernia

b Upside-down stomach

Gastroesophageal Prolapse

■ Definition and Clinical Aspects

Gastroesophageal prolapse is defined as the partial intussusception of the anterior stomach wall or greater curvature into the esophagus. Based on published reports, it is discovered in up to 8% of patients who undergo upper GI endoscopy.

Usually there is coexisting cardial incompetence, and an axial sliding hernia is often present (Fig. 3.**17**). Clinical complaints may include retrosternal pain, usually after a rise in intraabdominal pressure (coughing), as well as bleeding and transient incarceration.

■ Diagnosis

 Endoscopic diagnostic criteria
▶ Folds of stomach wall protrude into the distal esophagus during retching, appearing as a fungiform mass (Fig. 3.**18**)
▶ Prolapsed stomach occupies all or part of the esophageal lumen
▶ Detectable in the midesophagus and lower esophagus during endoscope insertion

Differential diagnosis
▶ The typical appearance is unmistakable.

Checklist for endoscopic evaluation
▶ Typical appearance of the prolapse
▶ Signs of reflux disease
▶ Cardial incompetence
▶ Hernia
▶ Bleeding at the gastroesophageal junction
▶ Retroflexed view: bleeding in the cardial region

Additional Studies
▶ None

Comments

The clinical significance of gastroesophageal prolapse is uncertain. Complaints may occur during coughing and other acts that raise the intraabdominal pressure.

3

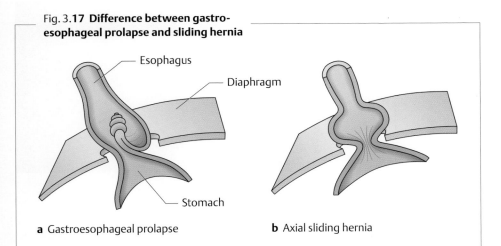

Fig. 3.**17 Difference between gastroesophageal prolapse and sliding hernia**

- Esophagus
- Diaphragm
- Stomach

a Gastroesophageal prolapse   **b** Axial sliding hernia

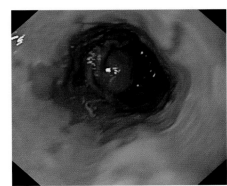

Fig. 3.**18 a–d   Gastroesophageal prolapse**

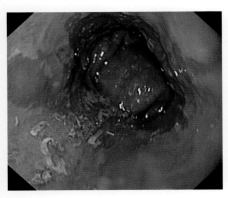

a

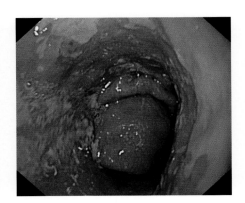

b

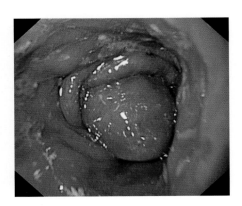

c

Mallory–Weiss Lesion and Boerhaave Syndrome

■ Definitions and Clinical Aspects

The Mallory–Weiss syndrome is characterized by bleeding from a mucosal laceration in the distal esophagus. The cause is a sudden rise in intraabdominal pressure, which may occur with forceful vomiting (especially in alcoholics), vigorous coughing, asthma attacks, or during pregnancy.

A complete rupture of the esophagus is known as Boerhaave syndrome. This complication leads to mediastinitis and has a high mortality rate. Mallory–Weiss lesions reportedly account for 10 % of all cases of upper gastrointestinal bleeding.

■ Diagnosis

Endoscopic diagnostic criteria

▶ Longitudinal blood-stained or bleeding tears (Figs. 3.**19**, 3.**20**)
▶ Located at the gastroesophageal junction
▶ Frequently posterior

Differential diagnosis

▶ Reflux esophagitis
▶ Typical history of Mallory–Weiss lesion: retching followed by bloodless vomiting, then vomiting of blood

Checklist for endoscopic evaluation

▶ Identify the bleeding source.
▶ Endoscopic hemostasis (see p. 155)
▶ Evaluate response.
▶ Complete esophagogastroduodenoscopy (EGD) to detect or exclude a concomitant bleeding source.

Additional Studies

▶ Oral contrast examination with a water-soluble medium (endoscopy is contraindicated in patients with a suspected perforation or if contrast extravasation occurs)
▶ Chest radiograph (pneumomediastinum is common in Boerhaave syndrome) (Fig. 3.**21**)

Comments

Treatment for a Mallory–Weiss lesion is described on page 155. Gastroscopy should be repeated after 24 hours. Boerhaave syndrome warrants early, aggressive surgical treatment.

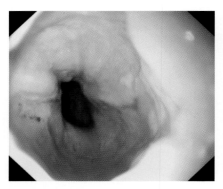

Fig. 3.19   Mallory–Weiss lesion
a   Forward view

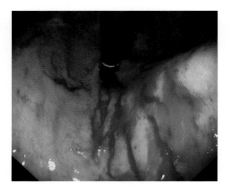

b   Retroflexed view

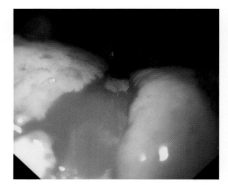

c   Close-up view

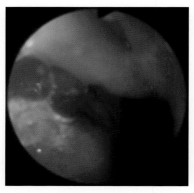

Fig. 3.20   Mallory–Weiss lesions
a   Small, blood-tinged mucosal tear in the area of the gastroesophageal junction

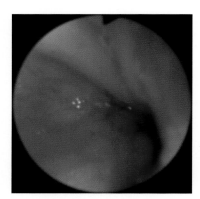

b   Mallory–Weiss syndrome

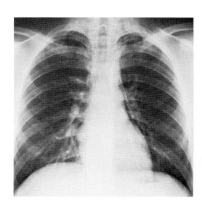

Fig. 3.21   Pneumomediastinum. Chest radiograph shows definite separation of the mediastinal pleura from the left cardiac border (from: Lange S, *Radiologische Diagnostik der Thoraxerkrankung.* Stuttgart: Thieme 1996).

Gastroesophageal Reflux and Reflux Esophagitis: Clinical Aspects

■ Gastroesophageal Reflux

Gastroesophageal reflux is a common endoscopic finding (Fig. 3.**22**). It is seen even in healthy individuals and usually causes no complaints. As a result, endoscopic detection does not necessarily indicate a pathological condition.

Pathophysiology. Because gastric juice contains substances that are corrosive to the esophageal mucosa, there are physiological mechanisms designed to protect the esophagus. Gastroesophageal reflux causes clinical complaints when these antireflux mechanisms fail. They include the sphincter mechanisms, the regenerative capacity of the esophageal epithelium, and the clearance function of esophageal motility, which curtails exposure to the corrosive gastric juice. Factors that predispose to gastroesophageal reflux are listed in Table 3.**2**.

■ Reflux Esophagitis

Reflux esophagitis refers to the gross or histological inflammatory changes that occur in the esophageal mucosa in response to reflux. The clinical picture is characterized by retrosternal or epigastric pain, heartburn, and dysphagia that periodically recur. Periods of remission with very mild clinical symptoms are followed by acute exacerbations. In many cases the complaints progress over time, eventually leading to complications such as chronic ulcers, scarring, strictures, columnar metaplasia, and adenocarcinoma.

Table 3.**2** **Pathophysiology of reflux disease**

Incompetent antireflux mechanisms
▶ Persistent increased transient relaxation of the LES
▶ Hypotensive LES
▶ Shortened LES
▶ Hiatal hernia
Impaired esophageal clearance
▶ Motility disorders (scleroderma)
Impaired gastric emptying
Volume and corrosiveness of the refluxate

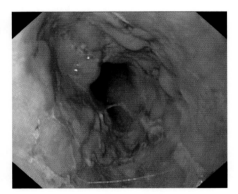

Fig. 3.**22** **Gastroesophageal reflux**

Complaints. A wide variety of complaints is possible, ranging from mild postprandial discomfort, which the patient may not even consider abnormal, to severe complaints like those seen in reflux esophagitis (Table 3.**3**).

Table 3.**3** **Symptoms of reflux disease**

Typical	Atypical
▶ Epigastric pain	▶ Vomiting
▶ Heartburn	▶ Chest pain
▶ Regurgitation	▶ Cough, "chronic bronchitis"
▶ Odynophagia	▶ Hoarseness
▶ Dysphagia	

Reflux Esophagitis: Diagnosis and Treatment

■ Diagnosis

 Endoscopic diagnostic criteria

▶ Involves the region from the distal esophagus to the Z-line
▶ Streaky pattern of spread, typically affecting the crests of mucosal folds
▶ Erythema, erosions, fibrin deposits (Fig. 3.**23 a–c**)
▶ Ulcerations (Fig. 3.**23 d**)
▶ Polypoid mucosal lesions (Fig. 3.**24**)

Differential diagnosis

▶ Carcinoma, especially in cases with marked inflammatory changes
▶ Mallory–Weiss lesion

Checklist for endoscopic evaluation

▶ Define and identify the lesion (erythema, erosion, ulcer).
▶ Location and extent
▶ Relation to incisor teeth and to gastroesophageal junction
▶ Pattern of spread of erosive changes (see Grading)
▶ Cardial incompetence or hernia?

▶ Signs of chronic changes such as scarring, ulceration, narrowing, ring formation (see Barrett Esophagus p. 70, Peptic Stricture p. 72)

Additional Studies

▶ 24-hour pH monitoring
▶ Esophageal manometry
▶ Radiographic contrast examination to detect or exclude a possible hernia not detectable by endoscopy

Comments

The diagnosis of reflux disease is based on the clinical presentation, endoscopic findings, histological examination, and 24-hour pH monitoring. It should be emphasized that the correlation between clinical complaints and endoscopic findings is poor. Also, there is not always a close correlation between endoscopy and histology, especially in forms with an essentially normal-appearing mucosa.

■ Treatment

▶ PPI therapy
▶ If unsuccessful: fundoplication
▶ Treatment of complications (see p. 157, 172)

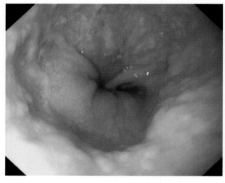

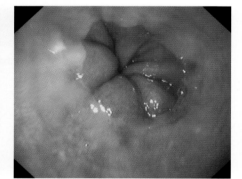

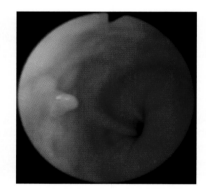

Fig. 3.23 Types of lesion that can occur in reflux esophagitis
a Mild, circumscribed erythema in the

b Streaky erythema

Fig. 3.24 Polyps in reflux esophagitis
a Reflux polyp at the boundary between the squamous and columnar epithelium

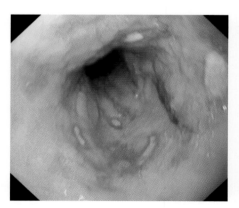

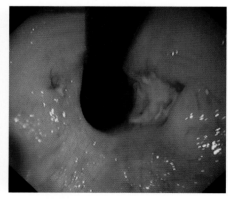

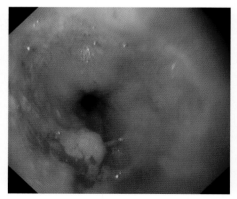

c Erosion

d Ulceration

b Reflux polyp

Reflux Esophagitis: Grading

■ Grade I–IV Reflux Esophagitis

The inflammatory lesions of reflux esophagitis are currently graded according to the Savary–Miller classification, which is summarized in Table 3.**4**.

Grades I–III. Grades I–III (Fig. 3.**25**) reflect a more or less pronounced acute attack. These grades may be complicated by superficial bleeding, but some cases initially resolve without sequelae.

Grade IV. Grade IV (Fig. 3.**26**) represents the chronic, complicated stage of reflux esophagitis, which is subject to its own dynamic. The most serious complications are obstructive strictures and adenocarcinoma secondary to columnar metaplasia of the esophageal epithelium.

Table 3.**4** **Endoscopic classification of reflux esophagitis, after Savary and Miller (1978)**

Grade	Endoscopic findings
I	One or more nonconfluent, longitudinal mucosal lesions with erythema and exudate
II	Confluent erosive and exudative lesions not covering the entire circumference of the esophagus
III	Erosive and exudative lesions covering the entire circumference of the esophagus
IV	Chronic mucosal lesions such as ulcer, stricture, and Barrett esophagus

Fig. 3.**25** **Grading of reflux esophagitis**

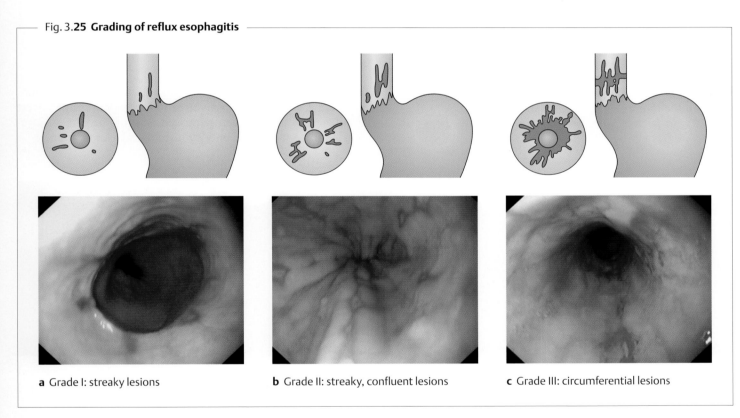

a Grade I: streaky lesions   **b** Grade II: streaky, confluent lesions   **c** Grade III: circumferential lesions

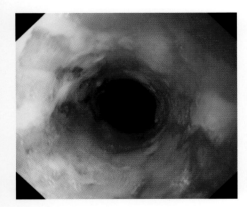
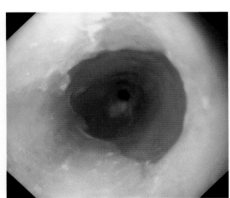
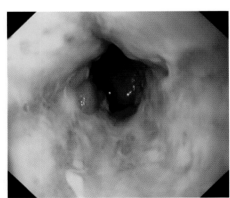

Fig. 3.26   **Grade IV reflux esophagitis**   **b** Barrett epithelium   **c** Peptic stricture
a Ulcer

Complications of Reflux Esophagitis: Barrett Esophagus

■ Definition and Clinical Aspects

In simple terms, Barrett esophagus is present when the squamocolumnar junction has migrated proximally into the esophagus by at least 3 cm (Fig. 3.**27**). This migration occurs when esophageal squamous epithelium that has been damaged by chronic reflux is replaced by metaplastic columnar epithelium.

This condition is found in up to 10% of patients with reflux esophagitis. The importance of the finding—and thus the necessity of identifying it, confirming it by biopsy, and monitoring its progression—lies in the approximately 10% risk of adenocarcinoma formation in the columnar-lined esophagus.

■ Diagnosis

 Endoscopic diagnostic criteria (Fig. 3.**28**)

▶ Reddened columnar epithelium lining the full circumference of the esophagus
▶ Squamocolumnar junction located at least 3 cm above the esophageal hiatus
▶ Frequent tonguelike extensions, occasional islands of epithelium
▶ "Short Barrett" = epithelial boundary shifted 2 cm proximally

Differential diagnosis

▶ Barrett carcinoma

Checklist for endoscopic evaluation

▶ Distance of the squamocolumnar junction from the incisors
▶ Location of the esophageal hiatus
▶ Epithelial islands in the proximal esophagus?
▶ Hernia?
▶ Incompetent cardia?
▶ Fresh inflammatory changes?
▶ Ulcer?
▶ Stricture?
▶ Neoplasia?

Additional Studies

▶ See Management

Comment

Barrett epithelium is frequently missed at endoscopy. Adenocarcinoma, which develops in up to 10% of patients with Barrett esophagus, is also frequently missed on gross inspection. Dysplasia can be diagnosed only by histological examination.

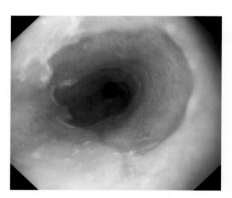

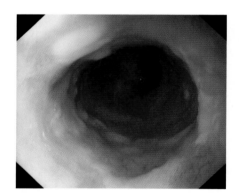

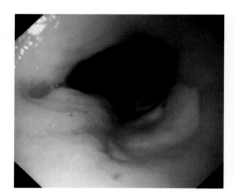

Fig. 3.28 Barrett epithelium
a The entire circumference of the distal esophagus is lined with metaplastic columnar epithelium

b The squamocolumnar junction has migrated to a level 32 cm from the incisors

c Barrett epithelium with ulceration

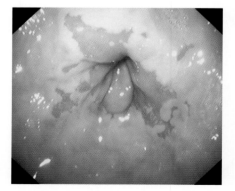

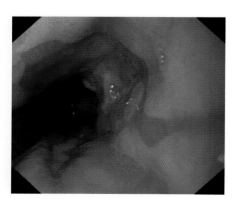

d "Short Barrett": the squamocolumnar junction has migrated by approximately 3 cm

e Early adenocarcinoma

Complications of Reflux Esophagitis: Management of Barrett Esophagus

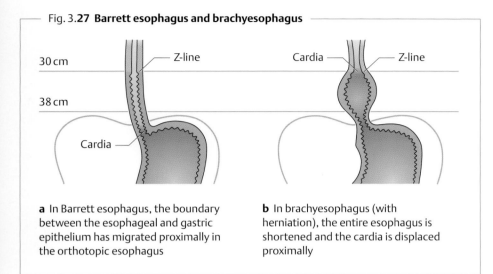

Fig. 3.**27 Barrett esophagus and brachyesophagus**

a In Barrett esophagus, the boundary between the esophageal and gastric epithelium has migrated proximally in the orthotopic esophagus

b In brachyesophagus (with herniation), the entire esophagus is shortened and the cardia is displaced proximally

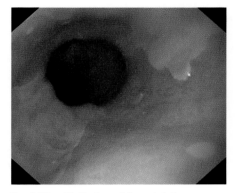

Fig. 3.**29 Methylene blue staining**
a Barrett epithelium prior to staining

■ Diagnosis

 Gross endoscopic criteria

▶ See page 70
▶ **Caution:** Barrett epithelium is often missed, as is adenocarcinoma, and it is very common to miss dysplasia at endoscopy.

Specimen collection

▶ Circumferential at various levels (every 2 cm)
▶ Methylene blue staining (see p. 178) (Fig. 3.**29**) and selective tissue sampling
▶ Brush cytology

b Areas with intestinal metaplasia are stained blue

Extended Testing

▶ Endosonography

■ Treatment and Follow-Up

▶ Barrett epithelium without dysplasia:
  – Yearly endoscopic follow-up with specimen collection
▶ Barrett epithelium with low-grade dysplasia:
  – 18-month follow-up
▶ Barrett epithelium with high-grade dysplasia:
  – Histological surveillance, then esophageal resection
▶ Alternatives:
  – Endoscopic treatment: thermal, photodynamic, mechanical

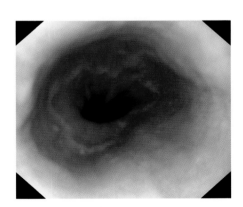

c Barrett epithelium

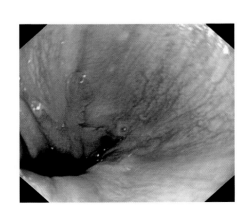

d Intense blue staining at the right edge ▷ of the epithelial tongue: intestinal metaplasia

Complications of Reflux Esophagitis: Peptic Stricture

■ Pathophysiology

Peptic strictures have a reported incidence of up to 15% in patients with reflux disease. Strictures develop as a result of longstanding gastroesophageal reflux and chronic, deep inflammation (extending into the submucosa) with fibrosis and scarring. They are found in the region of the gastroesophageal junction. Most strictures are short, but some may extend for several centimeters in the distal esophagus. The earliest change is usually a thickening of the Z-line, followed by concentric luminal narrowing that may later become eccentric and may be associated with a diverticulum-like outpouching of the esophagus proximal to the stricture.

■ Diagnosis

 Endoscopic diagnostic criteria (Figs. 3.**30**–3.**35**)

▶ Concentric or eccentric narrowing (Figs. 3.**30**, 3.**35**)
▶ Surface alterations
▶ Firm to the touch
▶ Pseudodiverticulum proximal to the stricture (Fig. 3.**32**)

Differential diagnosis
▶ Malignant stricture

Checklist for endoscopic evaluation
▶ Distance of the stricture from the incisors
▶ Extent
▶ Diameter (using biopsy forceps as a measure)
▶ Resistance to instrument passage
▶ Retroflexed view (Fig. 3.**33**)
▶ Gross evidence of malignant change?

Additional Studies
▶ Biopsy
▶ Cytology

Comments

A peptic stricture often requires endoscope treatment (see Dilation, p. 172).

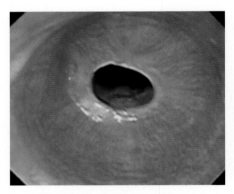

Fig. 3.**30** **Peptic stricture of the esophagus**

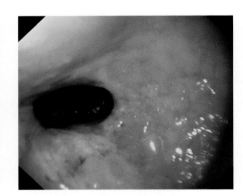

Fig. 3.**31** **Peptic stricture of the esophagus**

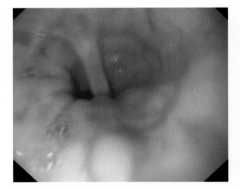

Fig. 3.**32** **Chronic reflux esophagitis.** Pseudodiverticulum proximal to the stricture

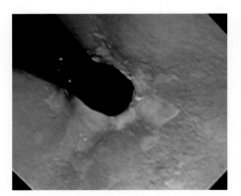

Fig. 3.**33** **Peptic stricture of the esophagus.** Retroflexed view

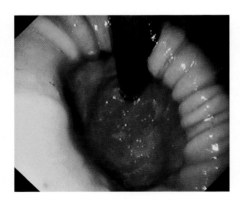

Fig. 3.**34** **Peptic stricture of the esophagus.** Retroflexed view

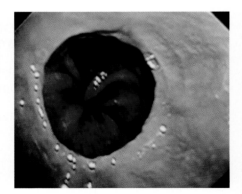

Fig. 3.**35** **Distal esophageal ring.** Most likely a result of chronic inflammatory changes. Fresh erythematous changes are also present

Candida Esophagitis

■ Pathophysiology

Infection with *Candida albicans* is the most common infection of the esophagus. It is frequently accompanied by *Candida* stomatitis. Predisposing factors are iatrogenic immunosuppression (chemotherapy, immunosuppression for organ transplantation, corticosteroid or antibiotic therapy), HIV infection, lymphoma, and diabetes mellitus.

■ Clinical Aspects

Complaints may be absent in early stages. Progression of the disease is marked by odynophagia, dysphagia, and retrosternal pain. The endoscopic diagnostic criteria are variable and depend on the severity and duration of the disease.

■ Diagnosis

 Endoscopic diagnostic criteria

▶ Location
  - All portions of the esophagus may be affected
  - Often located on the crest of the mucosal folds
▶ Morphology

Early (Fig. 3.**36a, b**)	– Scattered punctate plaques, which may be whitish, yellowish, or cream-colored
	– A few millimeters in size, slightly raised
	– Mucosa under the plaques may be normal, erythematous, or friable
	– Surrounding mucosa normal
Later (Fig. 3.**36c–e**)	– Streaky, confluent plaques and pseudomembranes
	– Tenacious, difficult to dislodge
	– Mucosa under the plaques is edematous, friable, bleeds easily
	– Mucosal erythema, erosion, ulceration, necrosis
Late (Fig. 3.**36f**)	– Changes affect the entire circumference
	– Luminal narrowing
	– Necrosis
	– Bleeding

Differential diagnosis

▶ The whitish plaques are fairly typical.
▶ Herpes simplex (HSV) esophagitis
▶ Cytomegalovirus (CMV) esophagitis

Checklist for endoscopic evaluation

▶ Morphology of the individual lesions
▶ Location and extent
▶ Signs of bleeding, ulceration

Additional Studies

▶ Brush cytology (often better than biopsy)
▶ Inspection of the oral cavity
▶ Radiographic contrast examination (may be normal)

Comments

Candida esophagitis is treated with fluconazole, and long-term prophylaxis may be advised. Most cases show good, prompt response. Repeat endoscopy is necessary only if there is no clinical response to therapy. Recurrence is common.

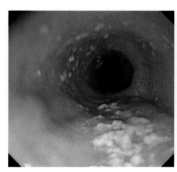
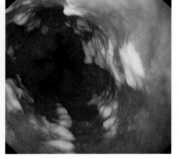

Fig. 3.36 *Candida* esophagitis
a Early stage

b Moderate involvement

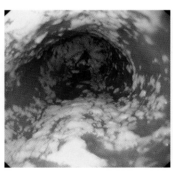
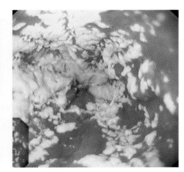

c Pronounced involvement

d Pronounced involvement

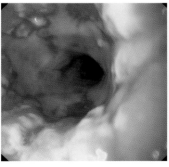
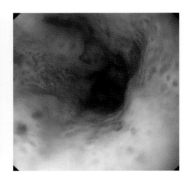

e Pronounced involvement

f Advanced form with thick exudate

Viral Esophagitis: Herpes simplex and Cytomegalovirus

■ Pathophysiology

Herpes simplex (HSV) and cytomegalovirus (CMV) esophagitis are less common than *Candida* esophagitis. They may coexist with it. Like *Candida* esophagitis, they occur predominantly in immunosuppressed patients, although herpes esophagitis can also occur in patients with a normal immune system.

■ Clinical Aspects

The symptoms are like those of *Candida* esophagitis. While all three forms of esophagitis have been described as having fairly typical endoscopic features, they cannot be distinguished from one another based on gross endoscopic criteria alone.

■ Diagnosis

 Endoscopic diagnostic criteria

▶ HSV: findings depend on the duration of the disease.
Early	– Vesicles
	– Normal mucosa between the lesions
Later (Fig. 3.**37**)	– Sharply demarcated ulcers with raised edges
	– Surrounding edema
Late (Fig. 3.**38**)	– Necrotic foci
	– Plaques
	– Confluent ulcers

▶ CMV
  – Large (1–3 cm), superficial ulcers with tonguelike extensions and maplike borders
  – Deep ulcerations, especially in HIV infections

Differential diagnosis

▶ *Candida* esophagitis

Checklist for endoscopic evaluation

▶ Morphology of the individual lesions
▶ Location, extent
▶ Signs of bleeding

Additional Studies

▶ Biopsy of margins (especially with HSV) and ulcer base for histological examination
▶ If necessary: immunocytochemical testing (HSV culturing, CMV)

■ Treatment

▶ HSV esophagitis
  – Aciclovir
  – Long-term prophylaxis, especially with HIV infection
  – Repeat endoscopy 10 days later
▶ CMV esophagitis
  – Ganciclovir, foscavir
  – Repeat endoscopy 10 days later

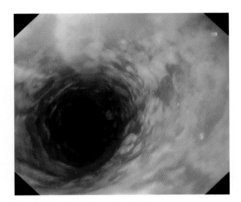

Fig. 3.**37**   **HSV esophagitis**

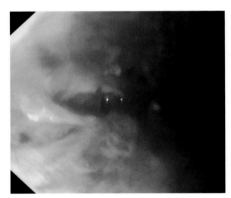

Fig. 3.**38**   **Viral esophagitis.** Necrotizing stage

Esophagitis due to Medications, Alcohol, or Foreign Bodies

■ Pathophysiology

Medications. Numerous medications can cause circumscribed lesions of the esophagus (Fig. 3.**39**). These lesions can result from several factors: the medication itself, its galenic properties, taking pills with an inadequate fluid volume, physiological and pathological constrictions, and motility disorders. The drugs that most frequently cause esophageal lesions include tetracyclines, penicillins, erythromycin, nonsteroidal anti-inflammatory drugs (NSAIDs), iron tablets, and potassium iodide.

Alcohol. Heavy drinking can cause patchy inflammatory erythema of the esophageal mucosa (Fig. 3.**40**). With abstinence, these changes are quickly and completely reversible.

Foreign bodies. Foreign bodies, including nasogastric tubes, can incite inflammatory changes through pressure injury and also by promoting gastroesophageal reflux (Fig. 3.**41**).

■ Diagnosis

 Endoscopic diagnostic criteria

▶ Medications (Fig. 3.**39**)
Location – Predilection for middle and lower third
– Aortic constriction
– Retrosternal esophagus
– Just above the distal constriction
Morphology – Isolated, sometimes confluent lesions, which may be on opposite walls ("kissing ulcers")
– Sharply circumscribed mucosal defects with punched-out appearance
– Erythema, erosion, ulceration, pseudomembranes
– Drug residues

▶ Alcohol (Fig. 3.**40**)
Location – Entire esophagus
Morphology – Circumscribed or diffuse erythema

Differential diagnosis

▶ Distal reflux esophagitis
▶ Esophageal carcinoma

Checklist for endoscopic evaluation

▶ Location (in centimeters and relative to constrictions)
▶ Size
▶ Depth
▶ Signs of bleeding?
▶ Detectable motility disorder?

Additional Studies

▶ None (history is important)

Comments

No specific treatment is available. The offending agent should be withdrawn.

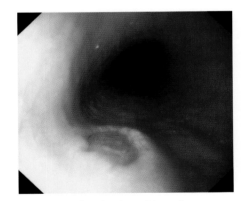

Fig. 3.**39 Ulcer in the midesophagus.** Medication-induced

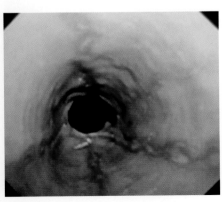

Fig. 3.**40 Streaky esophagitis due to heavy alcohol consumption**

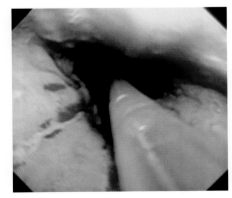

Fig. 3.**41 Esophagitis caused by an ind-welling nasogastric tube**
a Erosions

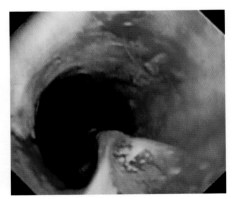

b Erosions and pseudomembranes

Alkaline Reflux Esophagitis and Radiogenic Esophagitis

■ Alkaline Reflux Esophagitis

Besides hydrochloric acid from the stomach, the esophagus can also sustain significant, clinically relevant damage from the reflux of duodenal alkaline secretions containing bile salts. This type of reflux is most commonly seen after gastrointestinal surgery, particularly a Billroth II gastroenterostomy.

■ Diagnosis

 Endoscopic diagnostic criteria (Fig. 3.42)

▶ Bile-tinged esophageal secretion
▶ Previously operated stomach
▶ Mucosal damage like that seen in peptic reflux esophagitis

Differential diagnosis

▶ Peptic esophagitis

Checklist for endoscopic evaluation

▶ Look for bile-tinged secretion
▶ Evaluate gastroesophageal junction
▶ Describe mucosal findings
▶ Determine extent of mucosal findings
▶ Identify postoperative anatomy
▶ Outflow obstruction?

Additional Studies

▶ Gastric juice sample for pH measurement
▶ Upper gastrointestinal contrast series: Reflux? Obstruction?

Comments

A trial of antacids or sucralfate is recommended. A prokinetic agent should also be administered.

■ Radiogenic Esophagitis

Radiotherapy for pulmonary and mediastinal tumors can induce esophagitis at doses as low as 30 Gy. The endoscopic findings depend on the extent of the irradiation and the timing of the examination.

■ Diagnosis

 Endoscopic diagnostic criteria (Fig. 3.43)

▶ Highly variable
▶ Acute:
  – Erythema, edema
  – Luminal narrowing
  – Sloughing, ulceration, necrosis, pseudomembranes
▶ Subacute and chronic:
  – Ulceration, fistulation
  – Strictures, whitish scars
  – Telangiectatic vessels

Differential diagnosis

▶ With a typical history, the diagnosis is reasonably certain

Checklist for endoscopic evaluation

▶ Location of the lesions
▶ Extent
▶ Severity of any strictures that are present

Additional Studies

▶ **Caution:** Biopsy poses a risk of fistula formation.

Comments

No specific treatment is available. Strictures may respond to peroral dilation.

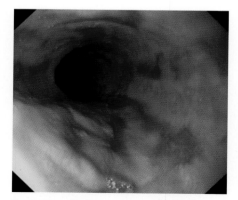

Fig. 3.42 **Alkaline reflux esophagitis in a postgastrectomy patient**

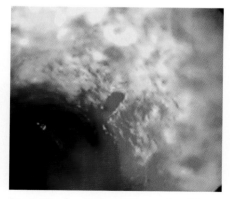

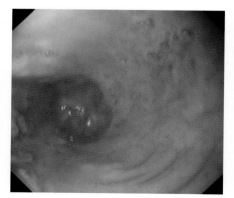

Fig. 3.43 a, b **Radiogenic esophagitis**   **b**

Esophagitis due to Corrosive Ingestion or Crohn Disease

■ Corrosive Ingestion

Chemical injury of the esophagus can be diagnosed from the patient's history. Initial treatment consists of prompt supportive care. The role of endoscopy lies in evaluating the extent of the injury. The examination must be done with extreme care due to the increased risk of perforation. Endoscopy should be performed within 12 hours of the corrosive injury, since postponing the examination will increase the risk of perforation.

■ Diagnosis

Contraindications to Endoscopy

▶ Perforation, peritonitis, suspected mediastinitis
▶ Necrosis in the hypopharynx, necrotizing epiglottitis
▶ Respiratory failure, shock

Studies Prior to Endoscopy

▶ Standing chest radiograph: pleural effusion?
▶ Plain abdominal radiograph, standing and LLD

 Endoscopic diagnostic criteria (Fig. 3.44)

▶ Early:
  – Erythema, diffuse or focal edema, blistering
  – Bleeding
  – Pseudomembrane, ulcer, slough
▶ Late:
  – Stricture
  – Fistula
  – Squamous cell carcinoma (caustic ingestion)

Differential diagnosis

▶ Endoscopic findings are easy to interpret in patients with a typical history.

Checklist for endoscopic evaluation

▶ Location of the injury
▶ Extent of the injury

Additional Studies after Endoscopy

▶ No tube placement
▶ Radiographic follow-up: Perforation?

Comments

The patient should be reexamined at three to four weeks, first with radiographs and then endoscopically.

Because caustic (alkaline) injuries are classified as premalignant lesions, endoscopic follow-ups should be scheduled once a year.

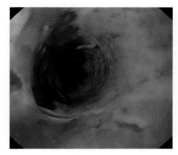 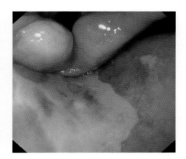

Fig. 3.**44** **Chemical-induced esophagitis**
a Lesions in the esophagus

b Corrosive lesions in the pharynx

■ Crohn Disease of the Esophagus

Crohn disease may affect the entire gastrointestinal tract, including the esophagus. Involvement of the esophagus alone is rare, however.

 Endoscopic diagnostic criteria (Fig. 3.45)

▶ Mucosal edema and erythema
▶ Nodular mucosa
▶ Ulceration and strictures

Differential diagnosis

▶ Viral esophagitis

Checklist for endoscopic evaluation

▶ Morphology of the individual lesions
▶ Location
▶ Number and size of the lesions

Additional Studies

▶ Biopsy
▶ Further standard tests for evaluating Crohn disease

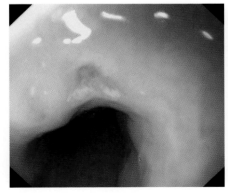 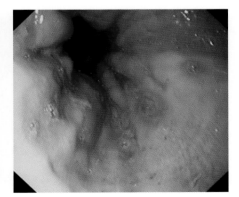

Fig. 3.**45 a, b** **Esophageal involvement by Crohn disease**

b

Synopsis of Inflammatory Lesions of the Esophagus

■ Clinical Complaints

The following complaints can result from inflammatory lesions of the esophagus:
► Heartburn
► Retrosternal pain
► Dysphagia
► Odynophagia
► Regurgitation

■ Causes of Complaints

Possible causes of the complaints should be briefly reviewed prior to endoscopy (Table 3.**5**). In many cases the history will greatly narrow down the differential diagnosis.

■ Differential Diagnosis

The main disease to be considered in differential diagnosis, from both a clinical and endoscopic standpoint, is esophageal carcinoma.

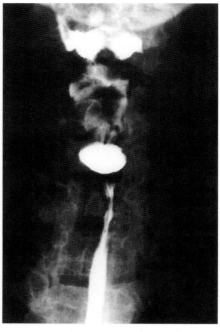

Fig. 3.**46**   **Oral contrast radiograph.** Lateral cervical diverticulum

Table 3.**5**   **Association between history and cause of complaints in various forms of esophagitis**

History	Cause of complaints
► Otherwise healthy	► Reflux disease
► Previous surgery – Billroth II stomach – Gastrectomy	► Alkaline reflux disease
► Known gastrointestinal disease – Inflammatory bowel disease – Motility disorder (scleroderma, achalasia)	► Crohn disease ► Stasis esophagitis
► Immunosuppression – HIV infection – Systemic hematological disease – Diabetes mellitus – Iatrogenic	► CMV, HSV, or Candida esophagitis
► Irradiation	► Radiation-induced esophagitis
► Ingestion of potentially harmful substances – Acute: medications, foreign bodies, alcohol – Prior history of caustic ingestion	► Pressure injury, toxic injury ► Esophageal neoplasia

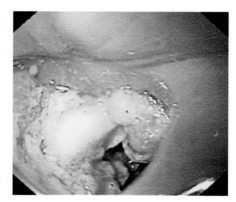

Fig. 3.**47**   **Cervical diverticulum.** Food residues in the diverticulum, compressing the esophageal lumen (top)

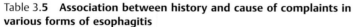

Diverticula: Definitions and Diagnosis

■ Definitions

Esophageal diverticula are more or less pronounced saccular protrusions of the esophageal wall. Traction diverticula (e.g., caused by extrinsic traction) affect the entire wall thickness (Figs. 3.**47**, 3.**48 b**), while in pulsion diverticula only the mucosa and submucosa protrude through a gap in the muscular wall (Fig. 3.**48 a**). There are three sites of predilection for diverticula in the esophagus: cervical diverticula (synonym: Zenker diverticula, comprising approximately 70% of all esophageal diverticula), thoracic diverticula (approximately 22%), and epiphrenic diverticula (approximately 8%).

■ Diagnosis

 Endoscopic diagnostic criteria

The endoscopic appearance depends on the size, location, and nature of the diverticulum (Figs. 3.**47**, 3.**49**).
▶ Cervical diverticulum
  Early – Small mucosal protrusion, which is often overlooked (stage I)
  Later – Deep pouch forming a "false lumen," whose axis is perpendicular to the longitudinal axis of the esophagus (stage II)
  Late   – Descent of the diverticular axis
         – Possible anterior displacement of the esophageal axis, with displacement of the diverticular axis into the original esophageal axis (stage III)
  –   May contain food residues

▶ Thoracic diverticulum
  – Location: midesophageal constriction, approximately 2 cm from the incisors
  – Small pouch (< 1.5 cm)
  – Shape: variable, often tent-shaped
  – May contain food residues
▶ Epiphrenic diverticulum
  – Location: 2–8 cm above the diaphragmatic hiatus
  – Small protrusion, usually in the posterior wall
  – Often coexists with axial sliding hernia
  – Occasional concomitant achalasia

Differential diagnosis
▶ Typical findings

Checklist for endoscopic evaluation
▶ Location (in centimeters from the incisors, physiological constriction, anterior/posterior)
▶ Size
▶ Contents
▶ With epiphrenic diverticula: Concomitant diseases? Hernia? Reflux? Achalasia?

Additional Studies
▶ Radiographic contrast examination
▶ With epiphrenic diverticula: manometry
▶ With thoracic diverticula: Tb testing, possibly computed tomography (CT)

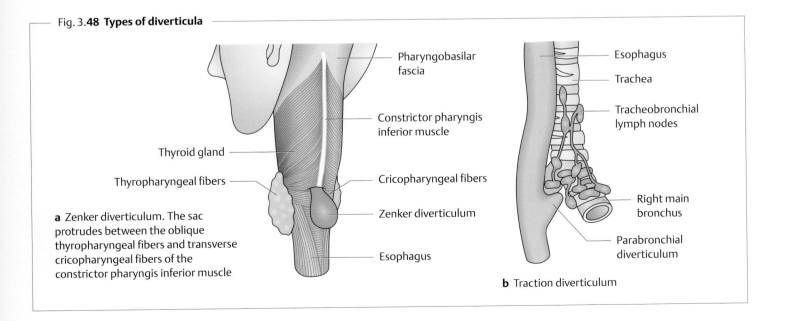

Fig. 3.**48 Types of diverticula**

Pharyngobasilar fascia
Constrictor pharyngis inferior muscle
Thyroid gland
Thyropharyngeal fibers
Cricopharyngeal fibers
Zenker diverticulum
Esophagus

a Zenker diverticulum. The sac protrudes between the oblique thyropharyngeal fibers and transverse cricopharyngeal fibers of the constrictor pharyngis inferior muscle

Esophagus
Trachea
Tracheobronchial lymph nodes
Right main bronchus
Parabronchial diverticulum

b Traction diverticulum

Diverticula: Details

■ Cervical Diverticulum

Cause. In a cervical diverticulum, the submucosal and mucosal layers of the esophageal wall protrude backward, usually slightly to the left, between the oblique thyropharyngeal fibers of the constrictor pharyngis inferior muscle and the transverse cricopharyngeal fibers of that muscle (Fig. 3.**48 a**). The cause is an abnormality of neuromuscular coordination in the upper esophagus combined with an anatomical weak point between the oblique and longitudinal muscle fibers.

Complaints. The earliest symptom is a foreign-body sensation. The generally progressive diverticulum then compresses the esophagus from behind, leading increasingly to dysphagic complaints. Large diverticula cause the aspiration and regurgitation of food residues.

Management. Endoscopy in this condition poses a considerable risk of perforation. Due to its progressive nature and the risk of aspiration, every cervical diverticulum should be evaluated for operative treatment.

■ Thoracic Diverticulum

Causes. Thoracic diverticula probably have diverse causes. A congenital anomaly with a persistent tissue bridge between the esophagus and trachea may have causal significance, as well as motility disorders and inflammatory wall changes (e.g., tuberculosis) in this region (Fig. 3.**48 b**).

Management. Thoracic diverticula are usually asymptomatic. There is generally no need for treatment.

■ Epiphrenic Diverticulum

Cause. Like Zenker diverticula, epiphrenic diverticula are believed to result from neuromuscular dysfunction at an anatomical weak point.

Complaints. Clinical symptoms may be mild, and heartburn is common. Epiphrenic diverticula are frequently associated with a hernia, achalasia, and spasms of the lower esophageal sphincter.

Management. Large, symptomatic epiphrenic diverticula should be treated operatively.

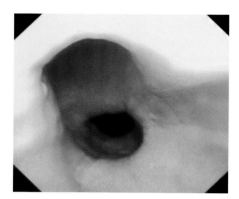

Fig. 3.**49 a–e**   Thoracic esophageal diverticula

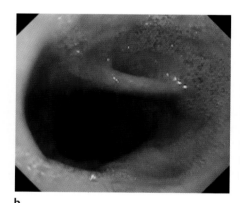

b

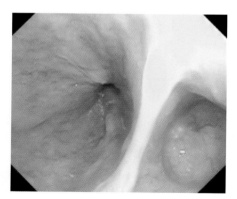

c

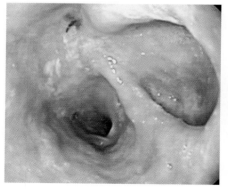

e

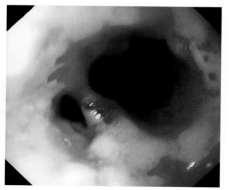

d

Achalasia: Clinical Aspects and Diagnosis

■ Clinical Aspects

Achalasia is a neuromuscular disease that causes dysfunction predominantly affecting the midesophagus and lower esophagus. It can lead to numerous complications.

Features. The essential features of achalasia are an absence of propulsive peristalsis in the midesophagus and lower esophagus and failure of the LES to relax with swallowing. The cause of the disease is ultimately unknown. On histological examination, inflammatory infiltrates are demonstrated in the Auerbach plexus.

Complaints. Complaints usually appear between 20 and 40 years of age, consisting initially of dysphagia for solid foods and later for liquids as well. Typical complications are chest pain, regurgitation, aspiration, and weight loss. Esophageal changes are characterized by a progressive dilatation over the nonrelaxing LES with the retention of food residues and consequent mucosal injury.

■ Diagnosis

One function of endoscopy is to confirm the diagnosis suggested by radiographs and manometry. A more important role is to exclude a malignant stricture by endoscopic biopsy. Radiographs cannot positively exclude a carcinoma of the cardia or distal esophagus. Moreover, achalasia itself is a premalignant condition with a long-term cancer risk of approximately 3%.

Studies and Measures Prior to Endoscopy

If achalasia is suspected or known to be present, or if fluid and food residues are detected in the esophagus at the start of endoscopy, the following measures may be indicated:
- ▶ Chest radiograph: mediastinal widening?
- ▶ Oral contrast study: dilated esophagus over the funnel-shaped constriction of the LES
- ▶ Fasting for 24 hours
- ▶ Any fluid residues are suctioned from the esophagus
- ▶ Examination may be aided by head-down tilt
- ▶ Use an endoscope with a large suction channel

 Endoscopic diagnostic criteria

- ▶ Early:
  - – Endoscopy may show no abnormalities
  - – Increased, "springy" resistance to instrument passage
  - – Failure of the cardia to open during prolonged observation (Fig. 3.**50**)
  - – Persistent rosette appearance
  - – Retroflexed view: cardia tightly closed around the endoscope
- ▶ Late (Fig. 3.**51**):
  - – Food residues and fluid in the esophagus
  - – Esophagus dilated, lax, elongated, tortuous
  - – Uncoordinated, nonpropulsive, or absent contractions
  - – Diverticulumlike pouch above the LES
  - – Increased resistance to cardial intubation
  - – Mucosal changes due to food retention: padlike thickening of the mucosa, erythema, petechiae, grayish–yellow deposits, rarely erosions, very rarely ulcerations

Differential diagnosis

- ▶ Malignant stricture (usually more difficult to intubate)
- ▶ **Caution:** A small cardia carcinoma may be missed in the forward view, so always inspect closely in retroflexion and take a generous tissue sample.

Checklist for endoscopic evaluation

- ▶ Evaluate the contents, shape, length, and course of the esophagus.
- ▶ Evaluate esophageal contractions.
- ▶ Observe, inspect, and evaluate the LES in forward and retroflexed views.
- ▶ Evaluate mucosal changes.

Additional Studies

- ▶ Oral contrast study: typical findings, see above
- ▶ Manometry: elevated pressure in the LES, absence of propulsive peristalsis
- ▶ Endosonography: thickening of the muscularis; detect or exclude cardia carcinoma

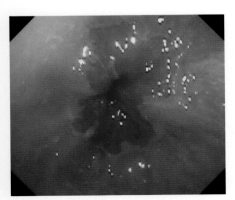

Fig. 3.**50** **Achalasia.** Sustained contraction of the LES

Achalasia: Treatment

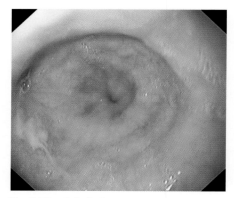

Fig. 3.51 Achalasia
a Marked prestenotic dilatation

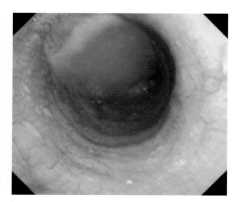

b Prestenotic pooling of secretions

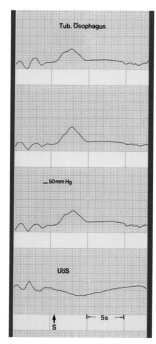

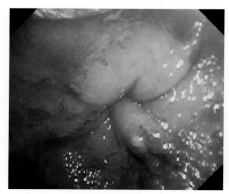

c Chronic inflammatory mucosal changes proximal to the stenosis

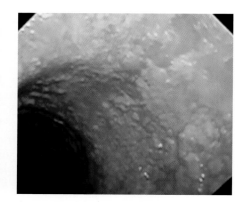

d Diverticulumlike dilatation proximal to the stenosis

Fig. 3.52 Manometric findings in hypomotile achalasia. The manometric traces show simultaneous hypotonic contractions in the tubular esophagus, with failure of the LES to relax with swallowing (from: Hahn and Riemann, *Klinische Gastroenterologie*. Vol. I, 3rd ed. Stuttgart: Thieme 1996)
les = lower esophageal sphincter
sw = swallow

■ Treatment Options

Symptomatic achalasia requires treatment.

Supportive Measures and Medications

▶ Supportive measures
- Small meals
- Chew thoroughly
- Do not lie down after eating
▶ Medications
- Nitrates, calcium antagonists

Medications cannot provide adequate long-term therapy.

Pneumatic Dilation

▶ Treatment of choice for symptomatic achalasia (see p. 172 f.)
▶ Two or three (up to five) dilations
▶ Complaints are relieved or significantly improved in over 70% of cases for more than one year and occasionally longer
▶ Perforation rate 1–3%

Surgery

▶ Indications
- Unsatisfactory response to multiple dilations
- Coexisting epiphrenic diverticulum
▶ Disadvantages
- Relatively high mortality (up to 3%)
- Postoperative gastroesophageal reflux in up to 40% of cases

Botulinum Toxin

▶ Still experimental
▶ Possible indications
- Unsuccessful pneumatic dilation
- High surgical risk
▶ Disadvantages
- Limited duration of response: two to six months (maximum: 24)
- Gastroesophageal reflux in up to 5% of cases

■ Follow-Ups

Due to the increased risk of carcinoma, endoscopy should be repeated once a year in patients with achalasia.

Diffuse Esophageal Spasm

■ Clinical Aspects

In diffuse esophageal spasm, normal peristaltic contractions occur along with irregular, synchronous, ineffectual contractions of the circular muscles (tertiary contractions), which can lead to regurgitation and retrosternal pain. Relaxation of the LES is not impaired (Fig. 3.**52**). The disease is very rare (incidence 0.2:100 000).

Complaints. Severe retrosternal pain occurs in brief episodes lasting only seconds. The pain is often triggered by drinking a hot or cold liquid but may also occur independent of meals, even during the night.

■ Diagnosis

 Endoscopic diagnostic criteria (Fig. 3.**54**)

▶ No typical endoscopic findings
▶ Some cases show segmental, irregular, nonpropulsive contractions leading to asymmetry of the esophagus
▶ Tenacious deposits and food residues are sometimes found
▶ The mucosa may appear normal

Differential diagnosis

▶ Examination artifact

Checklist for endoscopic evaluation

▶ Observe propulsive and nonpropulsive, synchronous segmental contractions
▶ Exclude a stenosing process

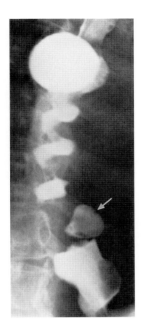

Fig. 3.**53 Diffuse esophageal spasm.** Oral contrast radiograph shows characteristic "corkscrewing" of the lower esophagus. A small pulsion diverticulum (arrow) and hiatal hernia are also present as incidental findings (from: Burgener, *Röntgenologische Differentialdiagnostik.* Stuttgart: Thieme 2000)

Additional Studies

▶ Oral contrast study: typical corkscrew or serrated contour during an attack (Fig. 3.**53**)
▶ 24-hour manometry: prolonged, synchronous contractions of high amplitude

Comments

Diagnosis is very difficult due to the paroxysmal nature of the complaints. The most rewarding study is manometry. Endoscopy is done to exclude other potential causes of the complaints, particularly malignant lesions.

■ Treatment

Diffuse esophageal spasm responds poorly to treatment. The patient should avoid drinking hot or cold liquids. A regimen of nitrates and calcium antagonists before meals may be tried.

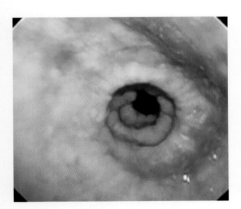

Fig. 3.**54 Diffuse esophageal spasm**
a Endoscopic appearance

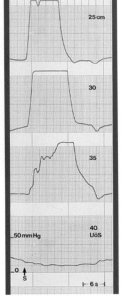

b Manometric findings in diffuse esophageal spasm. Simultaneous hypotonic contractions in the tubular esophagus. Normotonic resting pressure in the LES, which shows adequate relaxation with swallowing (from: Hahn and Riemann, *Klinische Gastroenterologie.* Vol. I, 3rd ed. Stuttgart: Thieme 1996)
les = lower esophageal sphincter
sw = swallow

Nutcracker Esophagus and Motility Disorders in Scleroderma

■ Nutcracker Esophagus

Nutcracker esophagus probably derives its name from the high-amplitude contractions that can generate intraluminal pressures of 150–400 mmHg. As in diffuse esophageal spasm, relaxation of the LES is not impaired. The cardinal symptom is chest pain.

■ Diagnosis

 Endoscopic diagnostic criteria

▶ No consistent endoscopic findings
▶ A spiral staircase-like pattern may be seen

Differential diagnosis

▶ Examination artifact
▶ Esophageal spasm

Checklist for endoscopic evaluation

▶ Observe and characterize peristaltic contractions.
▶ Exclude a stenosing process due to another cause.

Additional Studies

▶ Oral contrast study: may show nonspecific tertiary contractions
▶ 24-hour manometry: besides tertiary contractions, manometric traces consistently show high-amplitude directional peristaltic contractions of prolonged duration

Comments

This condition is also difficult to diagnosis due to its sporadic occurrence. A regimen of nitrates and calcium antagonists may be tried.

■ Esophageal Motility Disorders in Systemic Diseases: Scleroderma

Esophageal involvement is found in more than half of patients with systemic sclerosing diseases. Peristalsis and LES tonus are markedly diminished, allowing reflux of corrosive gastric juice. Other causes of impaired esophageal motility are diabetes mellitus, renal failure, neuropathies, and myopathies.

■ Diagnosis

 Endoscopic diagnostic criteria

▶ Signs of reflux esophagitis
▶ Strictures
▶ Rigid wall with no peristalsis
▶ Gaping LES

Differential diagnosis

▶ Reflux esophagitis
▶ Scleroderma
▶ Motility disorders secondary to diabetes mellitus, renal failure, neuropathy, or myopathy

Checklist for endoscopic evaluation

▶ Same as for reflux esophagitis
▶ Watch for peristalsis

Additional Studies

▶ Radiographic contrast examination
▶ Manometry
▶ 24-hour pH monitoring

■ Normal Variants

Besides the fairly well-defined pathological entities, it is common to find unusual motility patterns that cause no complaints and may be examination artifacts. They include fine, sawtooth-like contractions in the circular muscles of the esophagus and bizarre, propulsive contractions of the circular and longitudinal muscles. Rarely, the complete absence of peristaltic waves is noted in asymptomatic patients with normal-appearing mucosa.

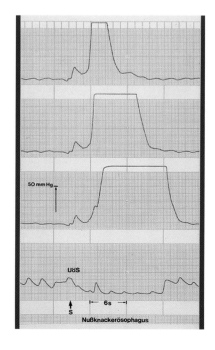

Fig. 3.**55 Manometric findings in nutcracker esophagus.** The traces show hypertonic propulsive contractions of prolonged duration in the tubular esophagus. The LES shows a normal resting pressure with adequate relaxation in response to swallowing (from: Hahn and Riemann, *Klinische Gastroenterologie.* Vol. I, 3rd ed. Stuttgart: Thieme 1996)
les = lower esophageal sphincter
sw = swallow

Esophageal Varices

■ Anatomy

Esophageal varices are distended submucous veins that project into the esophageal lumen. They are part of the collateral circulation that develops between the portal vein and vena cava in response to portal hypertension. They develop from the plexus of esophageal veins that drain into the azygos and hemiazygos veins. They receive blood from the left gastric vein and its esophageal branches and also from the short gastric veins via the splenic vein (Fig. 3.**56**).

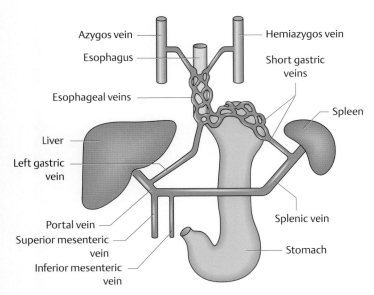

Fig. 3.**56** **Portocaval anastomoses in portal hypertension**

■ Clinical Aspects

Nonbleeding esophageal varices are asymptomatic. Rarely they are detected incidentally, but in most cases they are found during the work-up of liver diseases and occasionally in patients with acute upper gastrointestinal bleeding.

Bleeding. The most serious complication of esophageal varices is acute bleeding. Approximately 30% of all patients with varices have an episode of variceal bleeding. The mortality rate is 30–40%. The risk of rebleeding after an initial bleeding episode is 70%.

■ Diagnosis

 Endoscopic diagnostic criteria

The endoscopic appearance of esophageal varices depends on their grade (see p. 86) and the degree of air insufflation. Esophageal varices usually begin in the distal esophagus and may spread into the proximal esophagus with further progression (Fig. 3.**57**).

▶ Early:
  – Distended vein located at the level of the mucosa or raised slightly above it
  – May collapse when the esophagus is inflated with air
  – Affected vein may be bluish, grayish, occasionally whitish, or of normal color
  – One or more straight varices
▶ Later:
  – Varices project markedly into the lumen
  – Varices do not collapse completely in response to air insufflation
  – Tortuous, "string of beads", irregular calibers, may show circumscribed nodularity
▶ Late:
  – Occlude most or all of the esophageal lumen
  – Convoluted varices with nodular thickening
  – "Red signs" indicating a high bleeding risk (see p. 87)

Differential diagnosis

▶ Mucosal folds (Fig. 3.**58**)
▶ Dilated veins
▶ With circumscribed nodular varices: hemangioma, leiomyoma (Fig. 3.**59**)

Checklist for endoscopic evaluation

▶ Location and extent in centimeters from the incisor teeth
▶ Grading: size in millimeters and in relation to esophageal lumen
▶ Color, signs of high bleeding risk
▶ Shape: straight, nodular, convoluted
▶ Fundic varices? Hypertensive gastropathy?

Additional Studies

▶ Endosonography if findings are equivocal: varix, mucosal fold, hemangioma?
▶ Diagnosis of the underlying disease

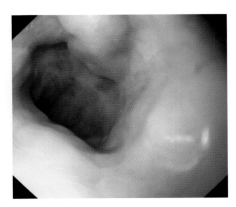

Fig. 3.**57** **Esophageal varices**

Esophageal Varices: Grading

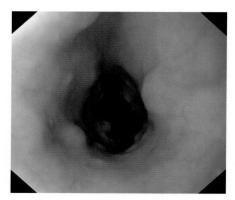

Fig. 3.**58** **Downhill varices.** Proximal esophageal varices secondary to upper inflow stasis

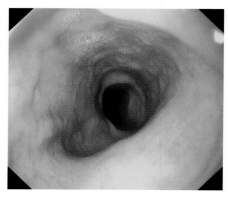

Fig. 3.**59** **Differential diagnosis**
a Mucosal folds

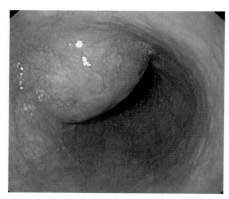

b Leiomyoma

Abb. 3.**60 Grading of esophageal varices**

The grades are based on size and luminal narrowing

I   Distended veins at the level of the mucosa

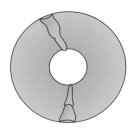
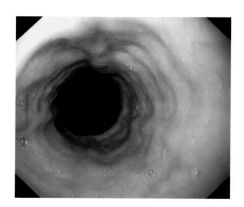

II Isolated, straight varices that project into the lumen with no significant narrowing (< 5 mm)

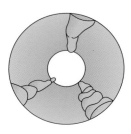
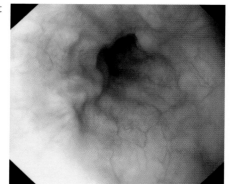

III Large, tortuous varices that cause significant luminal narrowing (> 5 mm)

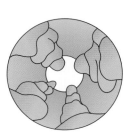
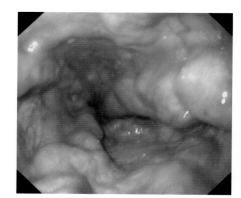

IV Almost complete luminal obstruction, signs of high bleeding risk

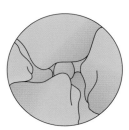
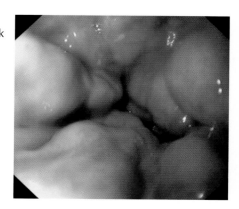

Esophageal Varices: Signs of High Bleeding Risk

■ Assessing the Risk of Bleeding

Location

▶ The farther proximal the varices extend, the more likely they are to bleed (Fig. 3.**61 a**).

▶ Concomitant fundic varices are associated with an increased risk of esophageal variceal bleeding (Fig. 3.**61 b**).

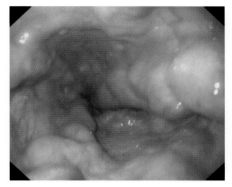

Fig. 3.**61   Signs indicating a high risk of bleeding from esophageal varices**

a Varices extending up into the proximal esophagus

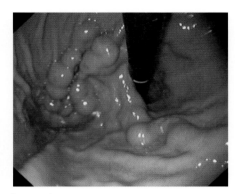

b Fundic varices

Shape, Size

▶ Small, straight varices rarely bleed
▶ Large, nodular, tortuous varices are prone to bleeding (Fig. 3.**61 c, d**)

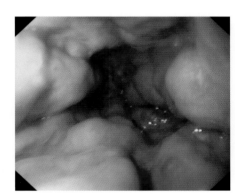

c Tortuous varices

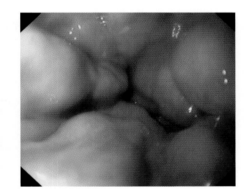

d Large varices

Color

The following indicate an increased bleeding risk:
▶ Diffuse erythema
▶ Dilated subepithelial venules on the varices:
  – Cherry-red spots (small, flat, red spots; Fig. 3.**61 e**)
  – Red wale markings (longitudinal red streaks; Fig. 3.**61 f**)
  – Hematocystic spots (larger, discrete, raised spots)

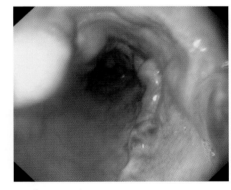

e Cherry-red spots

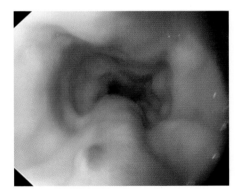

f Red wale marking

Other Signs

▶ Signs of reflux esophagitis increase the risk of bleeding (Fig. 3.**61 g**)

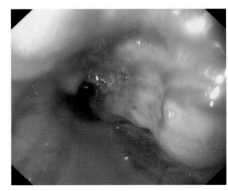

g Signs of reflux disease

3

Esophageal Varices: Treatment

■ Therapy

There are three instances when the endoscopist may be confronted with esophageal varices:

1. Before the first bleed
2. During the first bleed
3. After the first bleed

Treatment Before the First Bleed

The detection of esophageal varices before the first bleeding episode is generally accomplished during the staging examination for portal hypertension. Less commonly, the varices are detected incidentally.

Procedures

▶ It should be recognized during treatment planning that the prognosis depends more on the degree of hepatic insufficiency than on the severity of the esophageal varices.
▶ Mild varices do not require treatment.
▶ Pronounced varices with a high bleeding risk can be treated medically with 80–240 mg/day propranolol, which may be combined with 2 x 40 mg/day isosorbide mononitrate.
▶ Spironolactone in a dose of 100–200 mg/day can be considered as an alternative to beta-blockers.
▶ No endoscopic treatment
▶ No operative treatment
▶ No transjugular intrahepatic portosystemic shunting (TIPS) insertion

Treatment During the First Bleed

See page 147 ff.

Treatment After the First Bleed

The goal of emergency treatment is to control the primary bleeding and prevent rebleeding.

Procedures (Fig. 3.62)

▶ Esophageal varices are ligated or sclerosed with polidocanol. Fundic varices are obliterated with Histoacryl.
▶ In both cases, an initial second look is scheduled approximately four days after successful hemostasis.
▶ With good response to ligation or sclerotherapy, further follow-ups are scheduled at three weeks, three months, and six months.
▶ If the varices persist, sclerotherapy or ligation is continued at two- to four-week intervals with the goal of complete eradication.
▶ Small residual varices following primary ligation can be sclerosed.
▶ Propranolol may also be given as an adjunct.

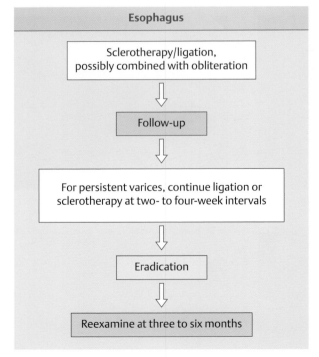
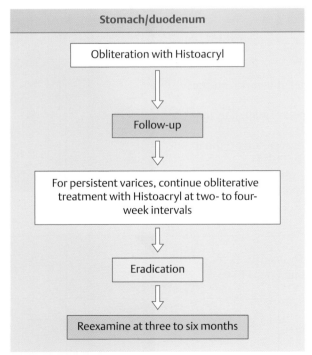

Fig. 3.**62** **Management of bleeding varices** (after Soehendra)

Esophageal Tumors: Overview of Benign Esophageal Tumors

■ Complaints

Esophageal tumors, whether benign or malignant, generally cause complaints only after they reach a certain size. Thus, they may be detected as incidental findings or, as is usually the case, as advanced tumors in symptomatic patients. The cardinal symptom is dysphagia. Bleeding is uncommon, even with large tumors.

The types of benign and malignant esophageal tumors are reviewed in Table 3.**6**. Extrinsic compression of the esophagus and esophageal varices should be considered in the differential diagnosis (Fig. 3.**63**).

Table 3.**6** **Benign and malignant esophageal tumors**

Benign esophageal tumors		Malignant esophageal tumors	
▶ Epithelial		▶ Epithelial	
– Papilloma	< 5 %	– Squamous cell carcinoma	> 80 %
		– Adenocarcinoma	< 15 %
		– Others	
▶ Nonepithelial		▶ Nonepithelial	
– Leiomyoma	< 70 %	– Leiomyosarcoma	< 5 %
– Lipoma, fibroma	< 15 %	– Kaposi sarcoma	
– Hemangioma	< 10 %	– Others	
– Granulosa cell tumors	< 5 %		

■ Differentiation of Benign Esophageal Tumors

Leiomyomas

Leiomyomas are the most common benign esophageal masses. They are usually found in the lower third of the esophagus and rarely cause complaints. Most are detected incidentally. They are located in the submucosa.

Lipomas, Fibromas, and Neurinomas

Lipomas, fibromas, and neurinomas are virtually indistinguishable from leiomyomas by their endoscopic appearance. They are very rare mesenchymal tumors.

Hemangiomas

Hemangiomas that are covered by normal mucosa are difficult to distinguish from leiomyomas endoscopically. Some, however, have a bluish tinge suggesting their vascular origin.

Papillomas

Papillomas are wartlike excrescences of squamous epithelium several millimeters in size. They are found predominantly in the distal esophagus. They are very rare.

Glycogenic Acanthosis

Glycogenic acanthosis is a frequent incidental finding with no clinical significance. The lesions consist of lentiform protuberances caused by the aggregation of enlarged cells with pronounced glycogen accumulation. This condition is of unknown cause.

■ Management

Most esophageal tumors are detected incidentally. Surgical treatment is indicated when clinical symptoms are present (dysphagia, bleeding) and for tumors that show marked enlargement or are larger than 5 cm, especially leiomyomas. A large leiomyoma can be difficult to distinguish from leiomyosarcoma, but its overall risk of malignant transformation is very low.

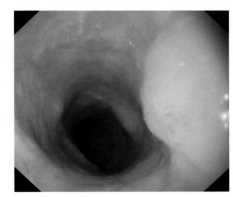

Fig. 3.**63** **Differential diagnosis of intramural tumors**
a Extrinsic indentation by a vessel or bronchus

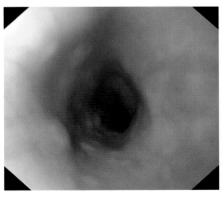

b Proximal (downhill) varices

Benign Esophageal Tumors: Diagnosis

 Endoscopic diagnostic criteria

- ▶ Leiomyoma (Fig. 3.**64 a**)
  - Well-circumscribed round or oval mass
  - Overlying mucosa is tense and intact, rarely ulcerated
  - Mucosa can be tented with biopsy forceps
- ▶ Lipoma, fibroma, neurinoma
  - Virtually indistinguishable from leiomyoma by their endoscopic features
- ▶ Hemangioma
  - Well-circumscribed mass covered by intact mucosa
  - Occasionally has bluish tinge
- ▶ Papillomas
  - Small, several millimeters in size
  - Raised, wartlike, hemispherical, sometimes flattened
  - Occur predominantly in the distal esophagus
  - Single or multiple
- ▶ Glycogenic acanthosis (Fig. 3.**65**)
  - Multiple, sometimes myriad, lentiform protuberances
  - Grayish–white
  - Occur predominantly in the distal esophagus

Differential diagnosis

- ▶ Leiomyoma: lipoma, fibroma, hemangioma
- ▶ Hemangioma: see above, also varices
- ▶ Papilloma: glycogenic acanthosis

Checklist for endoscopic evaluation

- ▶ Location
- ▶ Degree of luminal narrowing
- ▶ Circumferential extension
- ▶ Mucosal morphology

Additional Studies

- ▶ Biopsy: usually unsatisfactory for submucous tumors, even when several samples are taken at the same site ("dredge biopsy," "buttonhole biopsy").
  Caution: Biopsies can compromise a proposed surgical enucleation.
- ▶ Contrast esophagogram
- ▶ Endosonography: best study for determining the precise location of the lesion within the esophageal wall, differentiating between solid and vascular tumors, and detecting or excluding invasive growth (Fig. 3.**64 b**).

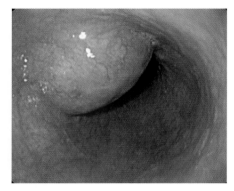

Fig. 3.**64   Leiomyoma**
a Endoscopic appearance

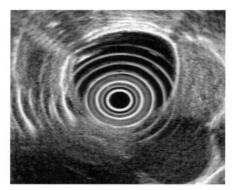

b Endosonographic appearance

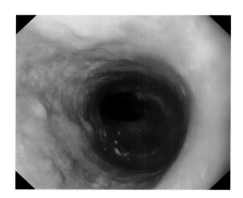

Fig. 3.**65 a, b   Glycogenic acanthosis**

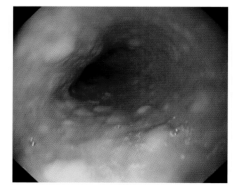

b

Malignant Esophageal Tumors: Diagnosis

■ Squamous Cell Carcinoma

The most common esophageal tumor is squamous cell carcinoma, which occurs predominantly in the middle and lower thirds of the esophagus. Predisposing conditions are nicotine and alcohol abuse, caustic injuries, achalasia, and the rare Plummer–Vinson syndrome (Table 3.**7**). The cardinal symptom is dysphagia, although even pronounced tumors may cause few if any complaints (Table 3.**8**).

Table 3.**7** **Risk patients and predisposing conditions for esophageal carcinoma**

> ▶ Alcohol abuse
> ▶ Nicotine abuse
> ▶ Caustic injury
> ▶ Barrett esophagus
> ▶ Plummer–Vinson syndrome
> ▶ Scleroderma
> ▶ Achalasia
> ▶ Palmar and plantar hyperkeratosis

Table 3.**8** **Symptoms of esophageal carcinoma**

▶ Dysphagia	90 %
▶ Weight loss	50 %
▶ Retrosternal pain	30 %
▶ Regurgitation	< 20 %
▶ Salivation	< 20 %
▶ Fetor	< 20 %

■ Adenocarcinoma

Adenocarcinomas account for less than 15 % of esophageal cancers, but their incidence is rising sharply. They may arise from ectopic gastric mucosa or columnar-lined esophagus, or they may result from the contiguous spread of a cardia malignancy.

 Endoscopic diagnostic criteria (Figs. 3.**66**, 3.**67**)

- ▶ Highly variable endoscopic appearance
- ▶ Early:
  - Superficial mucosal alteration, discoloration
  - Nodular or depressed mucosa
  - Erythema, erosion, or ulceration
  - Mucosa is friable, bleeds easily on examination and biopsy
- ▶ Late:
  - Exophytic, polypoid mass (most common form)
  - Fungiform, clefted surface, sometimes with central excavation
  - Erythema, erosion, ulceration
  - Pale gray, sometimes reddish discoloration
  - May be sharply or poorly demarcated from the surrounding mucosa

- Ulcerated carcinoma (second most common form)
- Deep ulcer with raised edges that show nodular thickening
- Diffusely infiltrating carcinoma (less common)
- Often shows circumferential growth, occasional submucous growth
- Indurated wall, eccentric luminal narrowing
- Surface may be nodular or ulcerated, but the mucosa may appear normal
- Contact with biopsy forceps shows a firm, submucous mass

Differential diagnosis

- ▶ Advanced esophageal carcinoma can almost always be identified as such on gross inspection.
- ▶ Early carcinoma requires differentiation from reflux esophagitis and pure, nonmalignant Barrett epithelium.

Checklist for endoscopic evaluation

- ▶ Location relative to the upper esophageal sphincter, aortic constriction, and cardia
- ▶ Distance of the upper and lower tumor margins in centimeters from the incisor teeth
- ▶ Type of growth
- ▶ Width of residual lumen
- ▶ Circumferential tumor extension
- ▶ Consistency
- ▶ Mobility of exophytic tumors

Additional Studies

- ▶ Biopsy with generous margins
- ▶ Chromoendoscopy (see p. 177 ff.)
- ▶ Endosonography
- ▶ Radiographic contrast examination
- ▶ Usual staging work-up

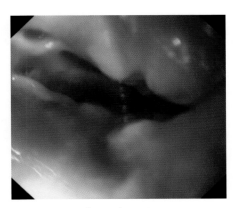

Fig. 3.**66** **Esophageal carcinoma**

Malignant Esophageal Tumors: Treatment and Follow-Up

■ Treatment

Surgery is the treatment of choice, although fewer than half of esophageal carcinomas are operable at the time of diagnosis. This accounts for the major importance of endoscopic palliation.

Endoscopic Palliative Treatment

The usual goal of endoscopic palliation is to restore an effective esophageal lumen, enabling the patient to swallow food and saliva. A less common goal is fistula closure. Various palliative treatment options are available (see p. 174 f.). The selection of a procedure should take into account the individual needs of the patient. It also depends on the experience of the endoscopist with different procedures. Percutaneous endoscopic gastrostomy (PEG) placement should be considered at an early stage, as in many cases it will eventually become impossible to pass an endoscope into the stomach.

Methods

Palliative endoscopic treatment options consist of laser therapy, bougie dilation, the implantation of a plastic endoprosthesis, and the placement of a self-expanding stent.

Laser therapy. The main drawback of laser therapy is that it is effective for only a few weeks. Also, it is not suitable for strictures involving a long segment of the esophagus.

Dilation and plastic endoprostheses. Bougie dilation and plastic endoprostheses have become superseded by self-expanding stents due to the high risk of perforation (up to 5%) and associated mortality.

Self-expanding stents. Coated or uncoated stents are advantageous in that they are relatively easy to insert, can be used even with high-grade tumor stenosis, have a relatively low complication rate, and are effective for a relatively long period of time. The folded metallic stent is introduced over a guide wire, usually under simultaneous fluoroscopic and endoscopic guidance, positioned within the esophageal tumor so that it overlaps the tumor margins, and deployed so that it can expand (see p. 174 f.). Problems and complications consist of displacement, perforation, pouch formation at the stent inlet, stent dysfunction due to tumor overgrowth, retrosternal pain, and mechanical mucosal injury at the distal end of the stent. Reflux can be a problem with stents placed in the cardia region.

Combined Radiation and Chemotherapy

Another palliative measure is combined radiation and chemotherapy, used for inoperable tumors or as a prelude to proposed surgery.

■ Follow-Ups

Postoperative follow-ups should be scheduled initially at three-month intervals and later at six-month intervals. CT is superior to endoscopy in detecting a local recurrence.

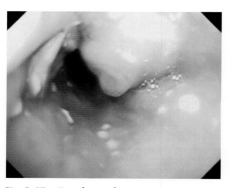
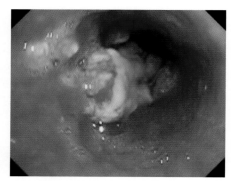
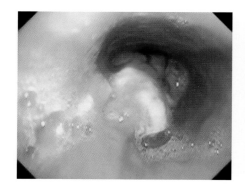

Fig. 3.**67** **Esophageal carcinoma**
a–e Squamous cell carcinoma

b

c

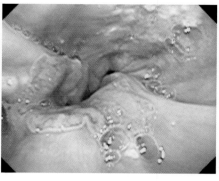

d

e

f Recurrent carcinoma

Postoperative Conditions

■ Type of Operation

Occasionally the endoscopist is confronted with postoperative changes in the esophagus. Usually this occurs after antireflux surgery and less commonly after resections. Endoscopy can define the postsurgical anatomical changes, their complications, and any recurrence of the underlying disease.

 Endoscopic findings

Antireflux surgery

▶ Endoscopic appearance, see page 126 (Fig. 3.**68**)
▶ Endoscopically detectable complications
  – Recurrence of reflux esophagitis
  – Wrap too tight

Esophagectomy, gastrectomy

▶ Endoscopic appearance
  – Gastric pull-up: demonstrate the anastomosis and the typical gastric mucosa distal to the anastomosis (Fig. 3.**69 a, b**)

  – Colon interposition: demonstrate the anastomosis and typical colon relief distal to it
  – Jejunal interposition: demonstrate the anastomosis and typical jejunal relief distal to it
  – Gastrectomy: demonstrate the anastomosis and small-bowel relief distal to it (Fig. 3.**69 c, d**)
▶ Endoscopically detectable complications in the distal esophagus
  – Erythema
  – Suture material
  – Erosions
  – Ulcerations
  – Cicatricial strictures
  – Recurrence of underlying disease

3

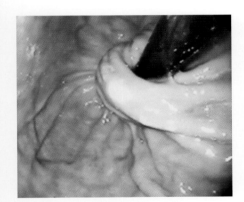

Fig. 3.**68** **Fundoplication**
a Typical endoscopic appearance

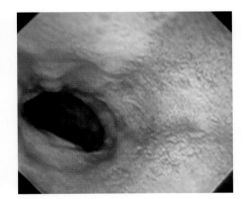

Fig. 3.**69** **Esophagectomy**
a Anastomositis following esophagectomy and gastric pull-up for esophageal carcinoma

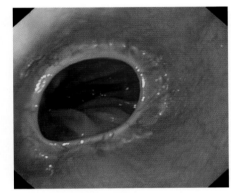

b View of the anastomosis following esophagectomy and gastric pull-up

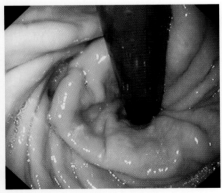

b Fundoplication performed as an antireflux procedure for reflux esophagitis

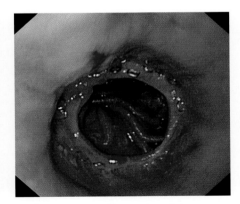

c Gastrectomy with esophagojejunostomy

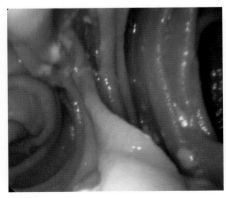

d Gastrectomy with esophagojejunostomy. View of the afferent and efferent limbs

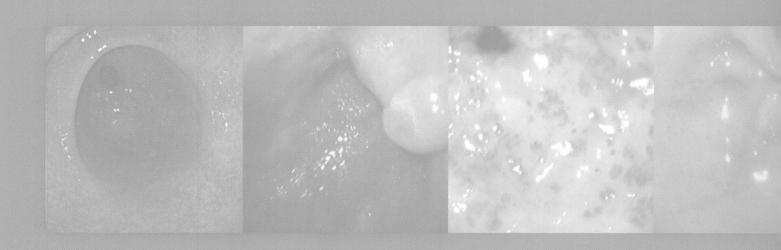

3.2 Pathological Findings: Stomach

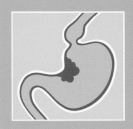

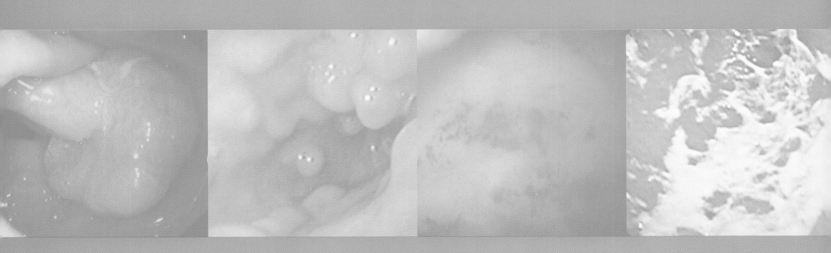

Overview of Pathological Findings in the Stomach

Table 3.**9** **Pathological findings in the stomach**

▶ Acute gastritis	▶ Portal hypertension
▶ Chronic gastritis	– Varices
▶ Gastric ulcer	– Hypertensive gastropathy
▶ Masses	▶ Postoperative changes
– Extramural	– Total gastrectomy
– Intramural	– Partial gastrectomy
– Epithelial	– Vagotomy and pyloroplasty
▶ Malignancies	– Fundoplication
– Carcinoma	▶ Rare findings
– Lymphoma	

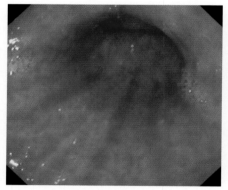

Fig. 3.**70** **Acute gastritis**

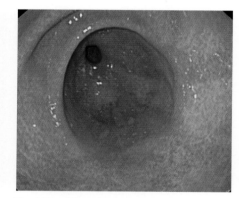

Fig. 3.**71** **Chronic gastritis**

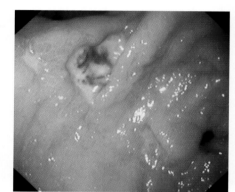

Fig. 3.**72** **Gastric ulcer**

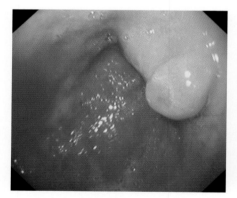

Fig. 3.**73** **Gastric polyp**

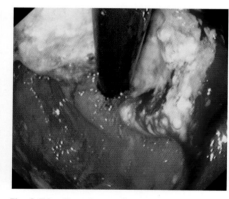

Fig. 3.**74** **Gastric carcinoma**

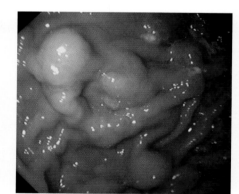

Fig. 3.**75** **Fundic varices**

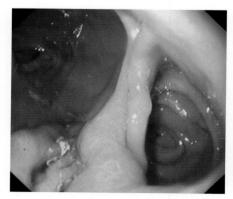

Fig. 3.**76** **Billroth II gastroenterostomy**

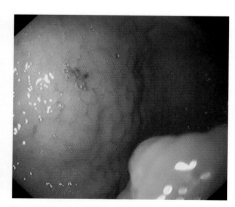

Fig. 3.**77** **Angiodysplasias**

Gastritis: Clinical Aspects

Acute and chronic gastritis are reactions of the gastric mucosa to various noxious agents. They are entirely different conditions, each presenting its own clinical, endoscopic, and histological features (Table 3.**10**). Both conditions, especially the chronic form, pose a special challenge to the endoscopist because the endoscopic findings correlate very poorly with the histological findings and clinical presentation.

■ Acute Gastritis

Acute gastritis can be caused by a variety of exogenous and endogenous agents (Table 3.**11**). More often than in chronic gastritis, endoscopy reveals signs that point to the correct diagnosis (Table 3.**12**; Fig. 3.**78**). The endoscopic features do not suggest a specific causative agent of the gastritis, however. The diagnosis of acute gastritis often relies on the clinical presentation (upper abdominal pain, anorexia, nausea, vomiting) plus the endoscopic findings, with histology showing little or no evidence of cellular infiltrate. The main role of biopsy is to distinguish between the various specific forms of gastritis (due to Crohn disease, infection, etc.).

Table 3.**10**   **Basic forms of gastritis**

▶ Erosive and hemorrhagic gastritis (acute gastritis)
▶ Chronic gastritis
▶ Special forms (specific gastritides)

Table 3.**11**   **Causes of acute gastritis**

▶ Bacteria (e.g., *Helicobacter pylori*)
▶ Medications (NSAIDs)
▶ Intoxication (alcohol)
▶ Reflux (stress)
▶ Trauma
▶ Mechanical lesion (foreign body, nasogastric tube)
▶ Vasculopathies
▶ Idiopathic

Table 3.**12**   **Endoscopically detectable features of acute gastritis**

▶ Edema
▶ Exudate
▶ Erythema
▶ Erosion
▶ Hemorrhage

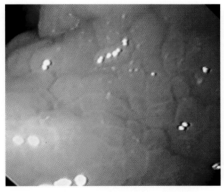

Fig. 3.**78**   **Endoscopic features of acute gastritis**
a   Marked edematous swelling of the mucosa

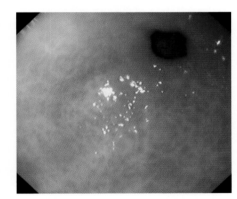

b   Exudate

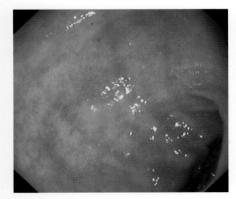

c   Erythema

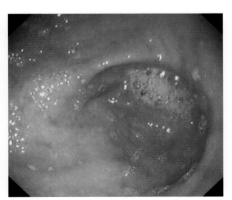

d   Erosions

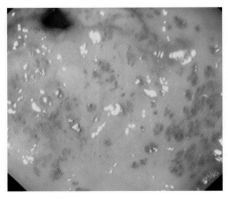

e   Hemorrhages

Acute Gastritis: Diagnosis

 Endoscopic diagnostic criteria (Fig. 3.**79**)

▶ Mucosa may appear normal in some cases
▶ Edema
  – Finely granular, bumpy surface
  – Prominent folds and prominent areae gastricae
  – Glassy, boggy appearance of the mucosa
▶ Exudate
  – Punctate, patchy, confluent deposits
  – Gray or yellowish streaks extending toward the pylorus
▶ Erythema
  – Punctate, mottled, confluent, or blotchy areas of erythema
  – On normal or reddened mucosa
  – Flat, sometimes slightly raised
  – Often found in the antrum
  – **Caution**: Redness alone is a very indefinite parameter.

▶ Erosion
  – Shallow epithelial defect in the mucosa
  – A few millimeters in diameter, sharply circumscribed; surrounding mucosa may be normal or erythematous
  – Thin fibrin coating usually present, occasionally fresh blood
  – Often found in the antrum, occasionally in the gastric body
  – Very reliable endoscopic criterion for acute gastritis
▶ Bleeding
  – Solitary or multiple petechiae, patches, or streaks, may be confluent
  – Red (fresh) or dark (hematinized)
  – Very reliable endoscopic criterion for acute gastritis

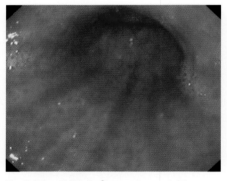

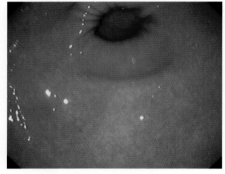

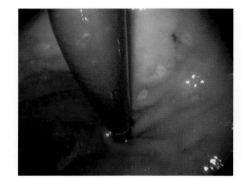

Fig. 3.79 Criteria for acute gastritis
a Streaks of erythema radiating toward the pylorus

b Mottled pattern of erythema in the antrum

c Erosions in the antrum

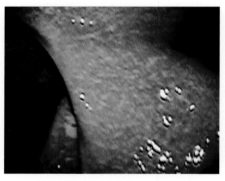

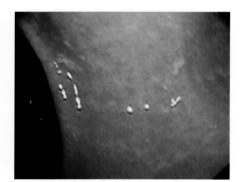

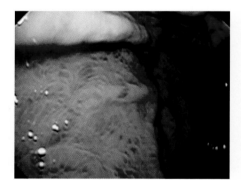

d–h Typical findings in acute gastritis

e

f

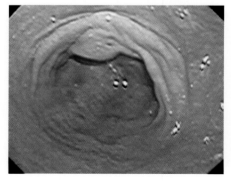

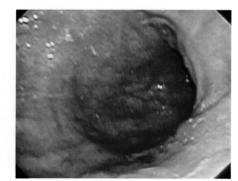

g

h

Acute Gastritis: Differential Diagnosis and Treatment

 Differential diagnosis (Fig. 3.**80**)

- Lymphoma
- Early carcinoma (circumscribed lesion)
- Chronic gastritis
- Hypertensive gastropathy
- Crohn disease
- Artifact

Checklist for endoscopic evaluation

- Morphology: morphology of individual lesions, distribution
- Location and extent: antrum, body, fundus, pangastritis
- Subjective grading of severity: mild, moderate, severe

Additional Studies

- Histological examination of biopsies taken from normal-appearing antral and body mucosa and from grossly abnormal mucosa
- Rapid urease test of biopsy specimens from the antrum and body

■ Treatment

Acute gastritis is often referable to a time-limited cause that can be identified in the patient's history (gastroenteritis, alcohol ingestion, medications, stress, etc.). Specific treatment is often unnecessary, but the offending substance must be avoided. Dietary measures are also recommended.

If medical treatment is needed, proton pump inhibitors (PPI) are used. Eradication therapy should be considered for severe cases of *Helicobacter pylori*–positive gastritis.

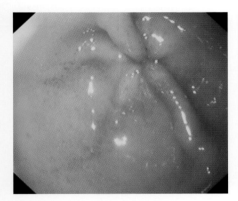

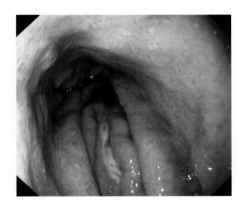

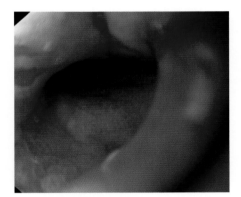

Fig. 3.**80** **Differential diagnosis of acute gastritis**
a Normal mucosa

b Crohn disease

c MALT lymphoma

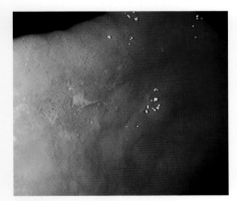

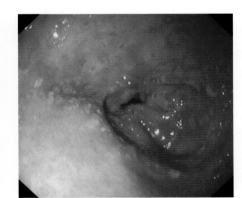

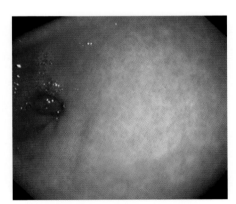

d Early-stage carcinoma

e Chronic gastritis

f Hypertensive gastropathy

Chronic Gastritis: Clinical Aspects and Classification

■ Clinical Features

Whereas acute gastritis is usually symptomatic and is responsive to dietary and pharmacological therapy, chronic gastritis frequently causes few or no complaints and shows a limited response to treatment (e.g., eradication therapy). The diagnosis of chronic gastritis can only be established histologically. There is no correlation between the endoscopic appearance and histological findings.

■ Classifications

In the past, numerous efforts were made to categorize the phenomenon of chronic gastritis. A widely used classification was based on etiological criteria, subdividing the disease into types A, B, and C. "Special forms" were added as a separate category (Table 3.**13**). Today a modified version of the Sidney classification (1990, 1996) is most commonly used. It takes into account etiological and histological parameters and the location of the gastritis (Table 3.**14**).

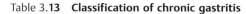

Table 3.**13** **Classification of chronic gastritis**

Type	Cause	Frequency
Type A	Autoimmune gastritis	approximately 5%
Type B	Bacterial gastritis	approximately 85%
Type C	Toxic chemical gastritis	approximately 10%
Special forms		

Table 3.**14** **Sidney classification of chronic gastritis**

Type of gastritis	Causative factors	Synonyms
▶ Nonatrophic	*H. pylori*, other factors	Type B gastritis
▶ Atrophic (Fig. 3.**82**)	Autoimmune process	Type A gastritis
– Autoimmune	*H. pylori*, nutrition,	Type B gastritis
– Multifocal atrophic	environmental factors	
▶ Special forms	Chemical irritation	Type C gastritis
– Chemical	– Bile reflux	Reflux gastritis
	– NSAIDs	NSAID gastropathy
– Radiogenic	Radiation-induced changes	
– Lymphocytic	Idiopathic, immunological, gluten-rich diet, medications, *H. pylori*	
– Noninfectious	Crohn disease	
– Granulomatous	Sarcoidosis, Wegener disease, vasculitides, foreign bodies, idiopathic	
– Eosinophilic	Food sensitivity, other allergens	
– Infectious (other than *H. pylori*)	Bacteria other than *H. pylori*, viruses, fungi (Fig. 3.**83**), parasites	

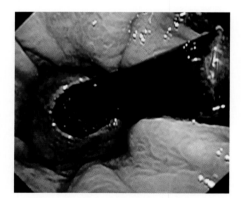

Fig. 3.**81** **Chronic gastritis.** Chronic inflammation with subtle histological findings

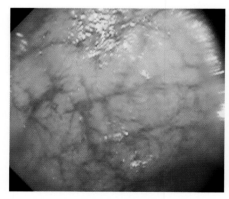
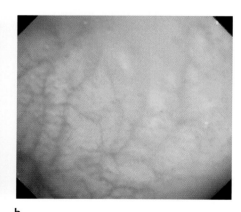

Fig. 3.**82 a, b** **Chronic atrophic gastritis**   b

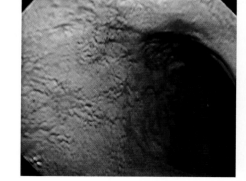

Fig. 3.**83** **Candidal gastritis in a patient with hepatic cirrhosis**

Chronic Gastritis: Diagnosis, Giant Fold Gastritis, and Ménétrier Disease

■ Diagnosis of Chronic Gastritis

 Endoscopic diagnostic criteria (Figs. 3.**81**–3.**86**)

▶ Endoscopic appearance does not correlate with histological findings.
▶ Possible endoscopic findings:
  – Possible absence of gross abnormalities
  – Edema
  – Erythema
  – Exudate
  – Hemorrhage
  – Shallow erosion
  – Polypoid erosion
  – Hypertrophic folds (type B gastritis)
  – Atrophic folds (type A gastritis)
  – Clearly visible submucosal vascular pattern (type A gastritis), especially in the body and fundus

Differential diagnosis

▶ Acute gastritis
▶ Early carcinoma (with circumscribed changes)
▶ Lymphoma

Checklist for endoscopic evaluation

▶ Lesion morphology (see above)
▶ Location: antrum, body, fundus, ubiquitous
▶ Subjective grading of severity: mild, moderate, severe
▶ Additional lesions: Ulcers? Hemorrhage?

Additional Studies

▶ Antral biopsy 2–3 cm from the pylorus
▶ Biopsy from the gastric body
▶ Biopsy from grossly abnormal areas
▶ Rapid test for *H. pylori*
▶ Antibodies against parietal cells (type A gastritis)
▶ Vitamin B$_{12}$ level (type A gastritis)

■ Giant Fold Gastritis

Giant fold gastritis refers to the presence of gastric folds more than 10 mm thick that are not effaced when the stomach is inflated with air. These folds are located in the body and fundus of the stomach. They are occasionally seen without discernible cause but also occur in the setting of *H. pylori* infection, Zollinger–Ellison syndrome, lymphoma, and Ménétrier disease.

■ Ménétrier Disease

Ménétrier disease is characterized by a hyperplasia of mucus-producing cells combined with gastric protein loss. Endoscopically, the rugal folds appear thickened and show increased tortuosity. Six-month endoscopic follow-ups are recommended initially, mainly to aid differentiation from lymphoma. Later, yearly follow-ups are scheduled due to the risk of malignant change.

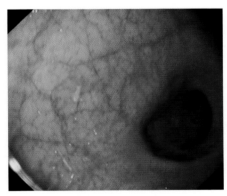

Fig. 3.84 Chronic gastritis. Prominent vascular pattern

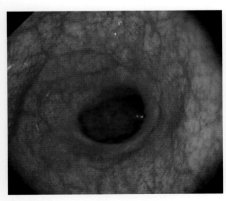
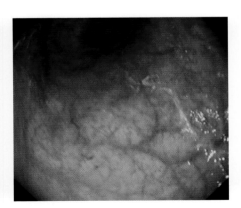

Fig. 3.85 a, b Mucosal atrophy in chronic gastritis

b

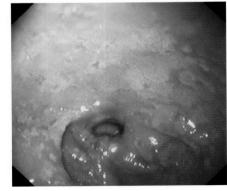

Fig. 3.86 Chronic gastritis. Histology: intestinal metaplasia

Gastric Ulcer: Clinical Aspects and Diagnosis

■ Definition and Pathophysiology

Gastric ulcer is an epithelial defect that penetrates the muscularis mucosae and extends into the submucosa.

Many precipitating factors have been identified, the most important of which are colonization of the gastric mucosa by *H. pylori* and the ingestion of nonsteroidal anti-inflammatory drugs (NSAIDs).

■ Clinical Features

There are no specific ulcer symptoms. Complaints range from immediate pain after eating and nonspecific epigastric discomfort to a complete absence of symptoms. The latter is particularly common with NSAID ulcers. Gastric ulcer is an endoscopic diagnosis, therefore. Endoscopy also allows tissue sampling to differentiate benign and malignant ulcers and permits *H. pylori* detection as a basis for causal ulcer therapy.

■ Location

Gastric ulcers can occur throughout the stomach. Eighty percent are located on the lesser curvature, usually in the antrum or at the angulus. The fundus, body, and greater curvature are less commonly affected. Basically any ulcer is suspicious for malignancy, and the likelihood of malignant transformation increases with the size of the ulcer. Multiple ulcers are usually seen in association with NSAID use.

■ Diagnosis

 Endoscopic diagnostic criteria (Figs. 3.**87**, 3.**88**)

The endoscopic appearance of an ulcer depends on its stage. Three stages are distinguished: active, healing, and scar:
► Active stage
  – Round, oval, linear
  – Bizarre shape

– Punched-out appearance
– Usually < 1 cm (**Caution:** easy to overestimate true ulcer size; measure with an open biopsy forceps!)
– Inflammatory swelling of the ulcer margin
– Ulcer base below the level of the surrounding mucosa
– Fibrin coating
– Greenish, yellowish, whitish
– Hematin
– Visible vessel: dark spot 1–2 mm in size
► Healing stage
  – Ulcer margin flatter and more irregular
  – Hyperemic mucosa grows from periphery to center
  – Fibrin coating on the ulcer base
  – Reddish mucosa covering the ulcer base
► Scar stage
  – Light spot
  – Atrophic mucosa
  – Folds radiating toward the scar

Differential diagnosis

► Carcinoma
► Lymphoma
► Crohn disease
► Boeck disease
► Eosinophilic gastritis
► Amyloidosis

Checklist for endoscopic evaluation

► Location: prepyloric, antrum, angulus, body, fundus, lesser curvature, greater curvature, anterior wall, posterior wall
► Size: novices tend to overestimate ulcer size. Estimate size with an open biopsy forceps.
► Number
► Shape: round, oval, linear, bizarre, irregular
► Ulcer margin: flat, raised
► Ulcer base: fresh blood, hematin, fibrin, visible vessel
► Assess need for endoscopic treatment. Stages I–IIa should be treated (see p. 145 f.).

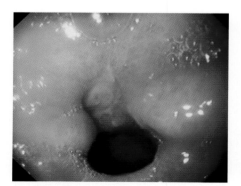 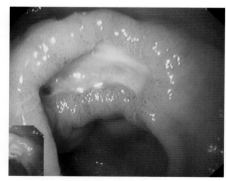 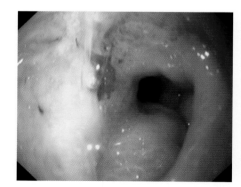

Fig. 3.87 Gastric ulcer
a Ulcer located just proximal to the pylorus

b Ulcer in the antrum

c Ulcer with an undermined margin

Gastric Ulcer: Management

Additional Studies

▶ Biopsy
  – Ulcer margin: one specimen per quadrant
  – Ulcer base: one specimen per quadrant
  – Ulcer center: one specimen
▶ Tests for detecting *H. pylori* (see p. 104)
  – Histological examination
  – Rapid urease test
  – Breath test
  – Serological testing
  – Culture method
▶ Radiography: Precede endoscopy with abdominal plain film if perforation is suspected.

■ Treatment and Follow-Up

Pharmacological Therapy

PPI are administered. If *H. pylori* is detected, the following regimen is used for eradication:

1. PPI, for example, pantoprazol, 40 mg 1–0–1
2. Clarithromycin, 500 mg 1–0–1
3. Amoxicillin, 1000 mg 1–0–1

Irritants, nicotine, and NSAIDs should be withdrawn.

Complications

▶ Oozing hemorrhage
▶ Massive hemorrhage (treatment, see p. 151 ff.)
▶ Perforation
▶ Gastric outlet stenosis

Follow-Ups

Endoscopy is repeated at four to six weeks, and new specimens are obtained. Additional follow-ups are scheduled according to the progression of healing.

Problems

▶ Refractory ulcer
▶ Dieulafoy ulcer (see p. 155)

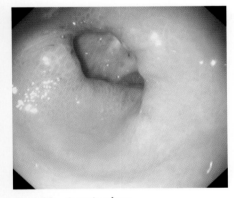

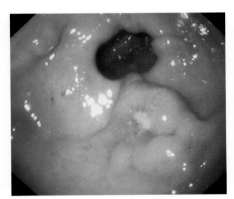

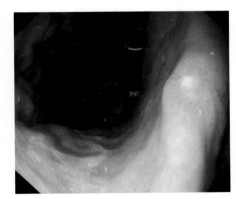

Fig. 3.**88** **Gastric ulcer**
a Ulcer in the antrum

b Ulcer with a fibrin coating

c Ulcers at the angulus

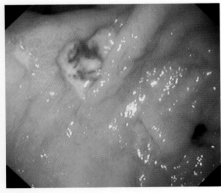

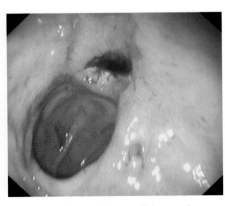

d Predominantly fibrin-coated ulcer with hematin traces

e Gastric ulcer with a small hemorrhage

Gastric Ulcer: Helicobacter pylori

■ Tests for Detection of Helicobacter pylori

Rapid Urease Test

Principle
- ▶ Based on the ability of the organism to convert urea into carbon dioxide and ammonia. A specimen of mucosa is placed into a test medium that contains urea and an indicator dye. If *H. pylori* is present, the pH rises, producing a characteristic color change, depending on the indicator used.

Sensitivity ▶ 90–95 %
Specificity ▶ 95 %
Advantages ▶ Economical
- ▶ Fast (15 minutes to three hours)
Disadvantages ▶ Does not indicate degree of inflammation
Evaluation ▶ Fast, simple, low-cost test to detect or exclude *H. pylori* colonization

Histological Detection

Principle
- ▶ Staining and direct histological identification of the organism in a tissue specimen (Fig. 3.**89**)

Sensitivity ▶ 85–95 %
Specificity ▶ 95–100 %
Advantages ▶ Standard method
- ▶ Provides information on inflammatory activity
Disadvantages ▶ Invasive
Evaluation ▶ Standard method

C$_{13}$ Breath Test

Principle
- ▶ The breath test, like the rapid urease test, is based on the ability of H. pylori to break down urea. The patient consumes a test meal containing C$_{13}$-labeled urea. The *H. pylori* urease splits the urea, and C$_{13}$-labeled carbon dioxide is exhaled. The exhaled air is collected and analyzed by mass or infrared spectroscopy.

Sensitivity ▶ 90 %
Specificity ▶ 95 %
Advantages ▶ Noninvasive
Disadvantages ▶ High cost
- ▶ Does not indicate degree of inflammation
Evaluation ▶ Ideal for confirming eradication

Serological Testing

Principle
- ▶ Serological tests are based on the detection of IgG and IgA antibodies against *H. pylori* in the serum. High titers of these antibodies are found during or immediately after a florid infection.

Sensitivity ▶ 85 %
Specificity ▶ 75–80 %
Advantages ▶ Noninvasive
Disadvantages ▶ Not useful for confirming eradication
- ▶ Relatively low sensitivity and specificity
- ▶ Does not indicate degree of inflammation
Evaluation ▶ Very useful for epidemiological studies
- ▶ Not useful for planning treatment or evaluating response

Culture Method

Principle
- ▶ It is possible to culture and identify *H. pylori* in special laboratories.

Sensitivity ▶ 70–90 %
Specificity ▶ 100 %
Advantages ▶ Can be used to test antibiotic sensitivity
Disadvantages ▶ Invasive
- ▶ Very costly
- ▶ Relatively low sensitivity
Evaluation ▶ Not a routine method, should be reserved for special investigations

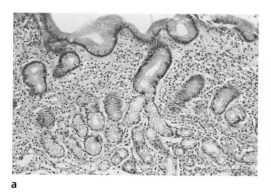

a

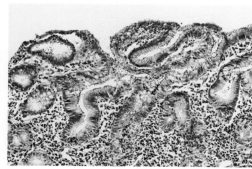

b

Fig. 3.89 Histological detection of H. pylori
a Low-grade, inactive gastritis
b With Warthin–Starry staining, even a relatively low-power view shows *H. pylori* organisms (black) densely colonizing the ridge summits and pit epithelium (from: Hahn and Riemann, *Klinische Gastroenterologie*. Vol. I, 3rd ed. Stuttgart: Thieme 1996)

Mass, Tumor, Malignancy: Overview

■ Classification

When distended by air insufflation, the stomach wall assumes a uniform appearance in which normal gastric folds are easily distinguished from the conspicuous mass effect produced by an extrinsic indentation, an intramural process, or a lesion in the mucosa (Table 3.**15**; Fig. 3.**90**).

Masses that bulge into the gastric lumen from the smooth or regularly folded surface often present the examiner with serious difficulties.
- ▶ The endoscopic diagnosis is frequently uncertain.
- ▶ The nomenclature of these changes, especially polyps, is confusing.

■ Role of Endoscopy

Endoscopy has a pivotal role in the definitive investigation of these findings.
- ▶ First the mass is visualized endoscopically and its morphology is described.
- ▶ Endoscopy makes it possible to obtain tissue samples, although some limitations apply (see Leiomyoma).
- ▶ Based on the endoscopic findings, the need for further testing is assessed. Endosonography is particularly rewarding in equivocal cases.

■ Synopsis

Table 3.**15** **Classification of masses in the stomach**

Indentations	Intramural processes	Polypoid lesions
▶ Sternum	▶ Leiomyoma	▶ Hyperplastic polyp
▶ Liver	▶ Hemangioma	
– Normal liver	▶ Lipoma	▶ Focal foveolar hyperplasia
– Metastasis	▶ Neurofibroma	
– Cyst	▶ Intramural gastric carcinoma	▶ Chronic erosions
▶ Spleen	▶ Leiomyosarcoma	▶ Elster glandular cyst
▶ Pancreas	– All of these intramural processes are indistinguishable by endoscopic examination!	▶ Adenoma
– Normal pancreas		▶ Ectopic pancreatic tissue
– Carcinoma		
– Cyst		▶ Carcinoid
▶ Duodenum		▶ Carcinoma
▶ Intraabdominal metastasis		▶ Lymphoma
		▶ Heterotopic Brunner glands

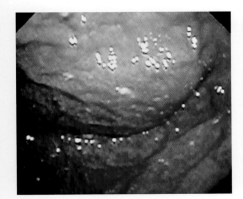 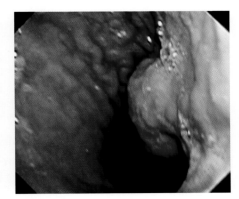 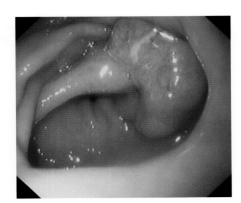

Fig. 3.90 Location of masses in the stomach
a Indentation of the stomach wall by an enlarged spleen

b Intramural mass

c Polypoid mass, in this case a gastric polyp

Mass, Tumor, Malignancy: Diagnosis

 Checklist for endoscopic evaluation

▶ Location
- Gastric region (cardia, fundus, body, antrum, prepyloric area)
- Specific site (lesser curvature, greater curvature, anterior wall, posterior wall)

▶ Size
- in millimeters or centimeters (estimate size with biopsy forceps)

▶ Shape and relation to substrate (Fig. 3.**91**)
- Flat, hemispherical, spherical
- Poorly demarcated, sharply demarcated, constricted base, pedunculated
- Pitted, irregular, cauliflowerlike

▶ Number

▶ Mucosal surface
- Normal-appearing, smooth, mobile
- Abnormal-appearing, reddened, fragile, fissured
- Glassy, glistening
- Ulcerated, eroded

▶ Relation to gastric wall (requires examination with biopsy forceps)
- Extramural indentation
- Intramural lesion
- Arising from the mucosa
- Mobility of the gastric wall
- Mobility of the mucosa

▶ Lesion morphology should permit a fairly accurate classification
- Indentation (extramural)
- Intramural lesion
- Polypoid lesion

■ Extrinsic Indentation

Organs that border the stomach tend to indent the gastric wall (see p. 48 ff.). The organs themselves—and to a greater degree, mass lesions affecting these organs—can produce circumscribed, tumorlike indentations in the stomach wall (Fig. 3.**92**).

 Endoscopic diagnostic criteria

▶ General
- Intact mucosa
- Mobility of the stomach wall over the indentation

▶ Sternum
- Typical location over the anterior stomach wall
- Identified by pressing on the abdominal wall below the sternum with the finger

▶ Spleen
- Typical location
- Large indentation located opposite the cardiac impression (see p. 51)

▶ Liver, hepatic metastases
- Located at the site of the hepatic impression in the anterior wall (see p. 50)
- Movement with respiration
- Intact mucosa

▶ Pancreas, pancreatic carcinoma, pancreatic pseudocysts
- Typical location in the posterior stomach wall at the body–antrum junction (see p. 49)

▶ Duodenum
- Sausage-shaped indentation in the gastric body or body–antrum junction
- Detectable peristaltic motion

▶ Intraabdominal metastases
- Located over the posterior stomach wall

Differential diagnosis

▶ Intramural process

Checklist for endoscopic evaluation

▶ See above

Additional Studies

▶ Endosonography

Fig. 3.**91 Nomenclature of polypoid mucosal lesions**

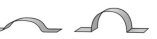
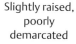
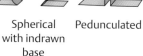

| Slightly raised, poorly demarcated | Hemispherical, moderately well demarcated | Spherical with indrawn base | Pedunculated |

Fig. 3.**92 Extrinsic indentation of the stomach wall**

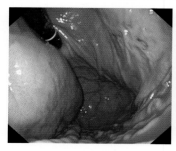
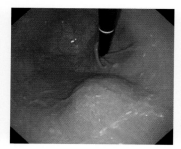
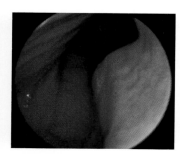
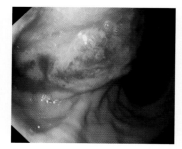

a Indentation of the fundus by an enlarged spleen

b Indentation by an hepatic metastasis

c Pancreatic process

d Penetration of a pancreatic pseudocyst into the stomach

Mass, Tumor, Malignancy: Intramural Tumors

■ Classification

Most intramural gastric tumors are detected fortuitously, but occasionally they are found during the investigation of gastrointestinal blood loss. The majority are mesenchymal neoplasms (leiomyomas, neurinomas, neurofibromas, lipomas). A smaller percentage are nonneoplastic, tumorlike polyps with intramural growth (heterotopic pancreatic tissue, Peutz–Jeghers polyp). Intramural tumors cannot be classified based on their endoscopic appearance, although the endoscopic findings (size, location) may suggest the nature of the mass.

Leiomyoma. Leiomyoma is the most common intramural tumor of the stomach (Fig. 3.**93 a**). Progression to leiomyosarcoma is considered rare and is most likely to occur with large tumors (>3 cm).

■ Diagnosis

 Endoscopic diagnostic criteria (Fig. 3.**93**)

▶ Hemispherical protrusion
▶ Small central depression may be present
▶ Mucosa intact or ulcerated (especially with large tumors)
▶ Mucosa can be lifted from the tumor (tented) with forceps due to the intramural tumor attachment.
▶ "Bridging folds" may be seen on opposite sides of the protrusion.

Differential diagnosis
▶ Extrinsic indentation

Checklist for endoscopic evaluation
▶ See page 106

Additional Studies

▶ Endosonography
▶ Cytological aspiration during endosonography
▶ Buttonhole biopsy: should be used very sparingly, as it can cause significant bleeding. Also, it is contraindicated if enucleation is planned.

■ Management Strategy

▶ Endosonography to exclude infiltrative growth
▶ Observation and follow-up
  – <2 cm
  – No malignant criteria
▶ Removal
  – >3 cm
  – Not definitely benign by endosonography
  – Hemorrhage
▶ Treatment of choice
  – Surgical enucleation

Fig. 3.**93 Intramural tumors of the stomach**

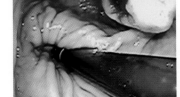
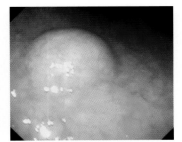

a Intramural leiomyoma with superficial mucosal ulceration

b Intramural lipoma

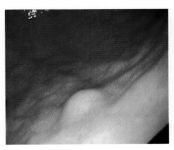
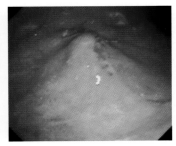

c, d Indeterminate submucosal mass in the stomach wall

d

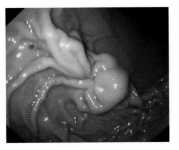

e Overgrown PEG tube, presenting as an intramural mass

Polypoid Lesions: Benign Tumors

■ Definition

The term "polyp" is used in different ways. To avoid misunderstandings, it will be used here as a purely descriptive term denoting a more or less circumscribed growth projecting into the gastric lumen from the level of the mucosa. The term itself says nothing about the origin, histological type (epithelial or mesenchymal), or biological behavior (benign or malignant) of the lesion.

■ Classification of Benign Gastric Tumors

Benign gastric tumors are found in approximately 3% of patients undergoing gastroscopy. More than 90% of these lesions are benign epithelial polyps. Mesenchymal polyps are rare.

As a rule, polyps are incidental findings that cause no complaints. Obstructive symptoms are rare, as is bleeding from superficial erosions or deeper necrotic foci. Only about 10% of polyps are classified as premalignant or show carcinomatous features on histological examination. Polyps may be isolated, multiple, or numerous. The term "polyposis" is used when the polyps number more than 20, or more than 100 according to some authors.

Table 3.**16** shows the classification of intramural and polypoid benign neoplasms, tumors, and polyps based on histological criteria.

Table 3.**16**   **Benign tumors of the stomach**

Neoplastic	Tumorlike
▶ Epithelial	▶ Nonneoplastic polyps
– Adenomas	– Glandular cysts
▶ Endocrine	– Hyperplastic polyp
– Carcinoid	– Peutz–Jeghers polyp
▶ Mesenchymal	– Inflammatory fibromatous polyp
– Leiomyoma	– Heterotopic Brunner glands
– Neurinoma	– Heterotopic pancreatic tissue
– Neurofibroma	▶ Special forms
– Lipoma	– Varioliform gastritis (= chronic erosions)
– Other rare forms	– Focal hyperplasia
	– Ménétrier disease
	– Other rare forms

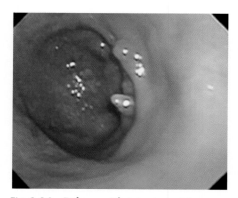

Fig. 3.**94**   **Polyps with intact gastric mucosa**

■ Frequency

Most of these diseases are rare or very rare. Reports on the distribution of the more common polyps vary considerably. The great majority of polyps consist of Elster glandular cysts in the gastric body, hyperplastic polyps, focal hyperplasias, and chronic erosions. Premalignant adenomas account for approximately 10% of polyps. The frequency data are summarized in Table 3.**17**.

Table 3.**17**   **Frequency of benign tumors of the stomach wall**

Benign tumor	Frequency
Elster glandular cysts	40–50%
Hyperplastic polyps	20–30%
Focal hyperplasia and chronic erosions	10–15%
Adenomas	ca. 10%
Heterotopic Brunner glands	<2%
Carcinoid	<2%
Heterotopic pancreatic tissue	<1%
Peutz–Jeghers polyp	<1%

■ Diagnosis

A confident diagnosis cannot be made from endoscopic findings alone. While it is often possible to make a diagnosis without histological evaluation, a biopsy should always be obtained if there is any doubt.

Polyps can be classified more accurately than intramural masses by their morphology, location, size, and number (see Checklist for endoscopic evaluation, p. 106).

> **Differential diagnosis of polyps and polypoid lesions based on morphological criteria**
>
> ▶ Mucosa intact
>   – Small hyperplastic polyp (Fig. 3.**94**)
>   – Small adenoma
> ▶ Mucosa altered, fragile, fissured
>   – Adenoma
>   – Carcinoma
>   – Large hyperplastic polyp
> ▶ Glassy, glistening mucosa
>   – Elster glandular cyst
> ▶ Hemispherical with depressed center
>   – Focal hyperplasia
>   – Chronic erosion
>   – Hyperplastic polyp with central erosion
>   – Early carcinoma
>   – Lymphoma
>   – Heterotopic pancreatic tissue
>   – Crohn disease
>   – Metastases

Polypoid Lesions: Differential Diagnostic Criteria

Differential Diagnosis of Polyps Based on their Location
(Fig. 3.**95**)

Polyp location as a criterion for differential diagnosis
(Fig. 3.**95**)

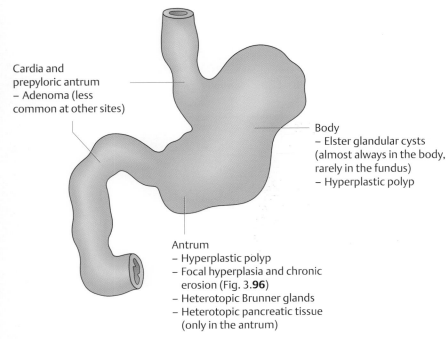

Cardia and prepyloric antrum
– Adenoma (less common at other sites)

Body
– Elster glandular cysts (almost always in the body, rarely in the fundus)
– Hyperplastic polyp

Antrum
– Hyperplastic polyp
– Focal hyperplasia and chronic erosion (Fig. 3.**96**)
– Heterotopic Brunner glands
– Heterotopic pancreatic tissue (only in the antrum)

Fig. 3.**95**   Polyp location as a criterion for differential diagnosis

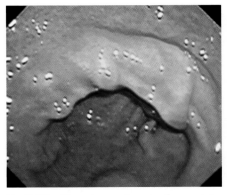

Fig. 3.**96**   **Chronic erosions in the gastric antrum**

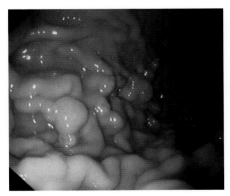

Fig. 3.**97**   **Elster glandular cysts in the gastric body**

Differential Diagnosis of Polyps Based on their Size
(Table 3.**18**)

Table 3.**18**   **Polyp size as a criterion for differential diagnosis**

Always < 1 cm	Usually < 1 cm
Focal hyperplasia Chronic erosion Elster glandular cyst	Ectopic Brunner glands
Often > 1 cm	**Very often > 1 cm**
Carcinoid Ectopic pancreatic tissue Hyperplastic polyp	Hyperplastic polyp Adenoma Peutz–Jeghers polyp

Differential Diagnosis of Polyps Based on their Number
▶ Almost always solitary
  – Adenoma
▶ Rarely multiple
  – Heterotopic Brunner glands
  – Heterotopic pancreatic tissue
  – Carcinoid
▶ Frequently multiple
  – Hyperplastic polyp
▶ Almost always multiple
  – Elster glandular cysts (Fig. 3.**97**)
  – Focal hyperplasia
  – Chronic erosions (Fig. 3.**96**)

Polypoid Lesions: Elster Glandular Cysts and Hyperplastic Polyps

■ Elster Glandular Cysts

Elster glandular cysts are among the most common polypoid lesions found in the stomach. They occur only in the gastric body and fundus and are often multiple. They do not grow and do not undergo malignant transformation.

 Endoscopic diagnostic criteria (Fig. 3.**98**)

▶ Occur only in the gastric body and fundus
▶ Usually < 5 mm
▶ Smooth, glassy, glistening
▶ Differential diagnosis
▶ Very typical appearance

Checklist for endoscopic evaluation
▶ See page 106

Comments

Usually the diagnosis can be established endoscopically. Elster glandular cysts are easily removed in toto with biopsy forceps. They are considered a harmless incidental finding.

■ Hyperplastic Polyps

Hyperplastic polyps are relatively common and are found throughout the stomach, with a predilection for the gastric body. They may be single or multiple and are usually no larger than 1 cm. Generally they show no growth tendency. They probably do not undergo malignant transformation in the gastric body, but there is a slightly increased risk of cancer developing elsewhere in the stomach.

 Endoscopic diagnostic criteria (Fig. 3.**99**)

▶ Occur in the gastric body and antrum
▶ Solitary or multiple
▶ Usually < 1 cm
▶ Spheroidal, sessile, occasionally pedunculated
▶ Mucosa usually appears normal, may be erythematous; small erosions sometimes occur

Differential diagnosis
▶ Adenomatous polyp
▶ See also page 109

Checklist for endoscopic evaluation
▶ See page 106

Comment

The diagnosis is established by histological examination.

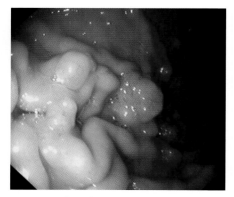
Fig. 3.**98 a, b** Elster glandular cysts

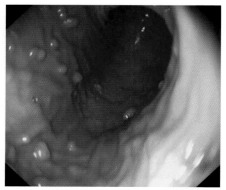
b

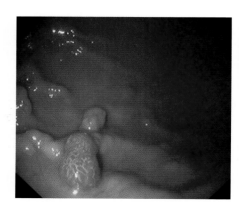
Fig. 3.**99 a, b** Gastric polyps

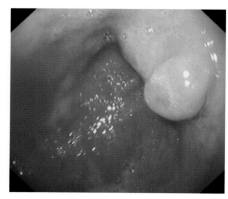
b

Polypoid Lesions: Focal Hyperplasia and Chronic Erosions

■ Focal Hyperplasia

Focal hyperplasias are a pathogenetically diverse group of polypoid mucosal changes that many authors do not classify as polyps (Fig. 3.**100**). They are found in association with chronic erosions, scars, and anastomoses. They are not considered a precursor of gastric cancer. *H. pylori*–associated gastritis is usually present.

 Endoscopic diagnostic criteria (Fig. 3.**100**)

▶ Predominantly in the antrum
▶ Multiple
▶ "String of beads" configuration
▶ Central depression

Differential diagnosis

▶ Chronic erosions
▶ See also page 109

Checklist for endoscopic evaluation

▶ See page 106

Additional Studies

▶ Tests for detecting *H. pylori* (see p. 104)

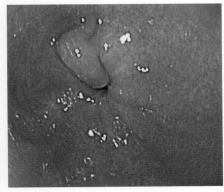

Fig. 3.**100** **Focal hyperplasia.** Polypoid outgrowth of mucosa in gastritis

■ Chronic Erosions

Chronic erosions are usually found in the antrum and less commonly in the gastric body. Reportedly, they can persist for months without change. Occasionally they are found in association with other morphological signs of gastritis but may also occur in asymptomatic patients with otherwise normal gastric mucosa. The endoscopic appearance is very typical.

 Endoscopic diagnostic criteria (Fig. 3.**101**)

▶ Size: 5–10 mm; circumscribed, resemble sessile polyps
▶ Central depression, usually fibrin-coated, rarely with traces of hematin
▶ Inflammatory border, thickened gastric folds in some cases
▶ Single, multiple, or numerous
▶ Occasional "string of beads" arrangement tracking toward the pylorus: "varioliform gastritis"

Differential diagnosis

▶ See page 109
▶ Specific lesions
  – Eroded polyps
  – Metastases
  – Lymphoma
  – Ectopic pancreatic tissue
  – Early gastric carcinoma
  – Crohn disease

Checklist for endoscopic evaluation

▶ See page 106

Additional Studies

▶ Unnecessary in most cases
▶ Biopsy if doubt exists

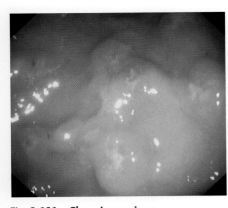 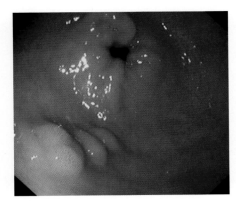 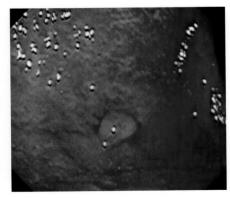

Fig. 3.**101** **Chronic erosions**
a Chronic erosions in the antrum

b "String of beads" erosions directed toward the pylorus

c Chronic erosion

Polypoid Lesions: Adenoma and Rare Findings

■ Adenoma

While relatively rare, gastric adenomas have a tendency to undergo malignant change. The frequency of the adenoma-to-carcinoma sequence is uncertain, however. Reportedly, carcinoma develops in up to 40% of patients with gastric adenomas larger than 2 cm.

 Endoscopic diagnostic criteria (Fig. 3.**102**)

▶ Most commonly located in the prepyloric antrum or near the cardia
▶ Size: 1–2 (up to 4) cm
▶ Surface irregular, septated, erythematous
▶ May show erosion or ulceration
▶ Mucosal erythema

Differential diagnosis
▶ See page 109
▶ In particular: hyperplastic polyps

Checklist for endoscopic evaluation
▶ See page 106

Additional Studies
▶ Biopsy

Comments
Gastric adenoma is a precancerous lesion. Endoscopic biopsy surveillance is adequate for lesions smaller than 1 cm. Lesions larger than 1 cm should be removed.

■ Heterotopic Brunner Glands

This is a rare condition seen predominantly in the gastric antrum (Fig. 3.**103 a, b**). The lesions are usually small (< 1 cm).

■ Carcinoid

Carcinoids may present as polypoid lesions. Occurrence in the stomach is very rare.

■ Heterotopic Pancreatic Tissue

Heterotopic pancreas is very rare and is found only in the antrum. The lesion is moderately large, occasionally exceeding 1 cm in size.

■ Peutz–Jeghers Syndrome

Peutz–Jeghers syndrome is an autosomal dominant condition characterized by perioral melanin pigmentation and intestinal polyposis. The polyps occur mainly in the small bowel and colon but may also be found in the stomach (Fig. 3.**103 c**). Histologically, the lesions are submucosal hamartomas that are usually 1–2 cm in size but may grow considerably larger. There is no risk of malignant transformation, but the risk of colon cancer is increased due to a greater frequency of adenoma occurrence.

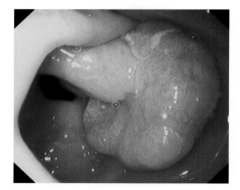
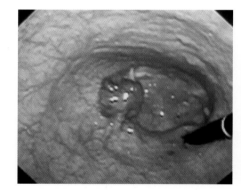

Fig. 3.**102** **Adenomas**
a Pedunculated gastric polyp. Histology: adenoma

b Gastric polyp. Histology: adenoma

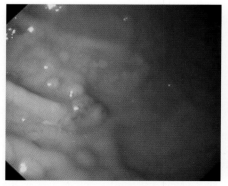
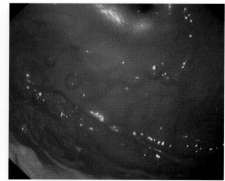
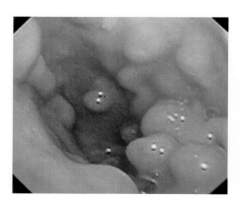

Fig. 3.**103** **Rare benign tumors of the stomach**
a, b Heterotopic Brunner glands

b

c Gastric polyposis in Peutz–Jeghers syndrome

Polypoid Lesions: Management

■ Treatment and Follow-Up

For polyps smaller than 1 cm, further management is contingent upon biopsy findings (Figs. 3.**104**, 3.**105**). Complete removal is indicated for polyps larger than 1 cm.

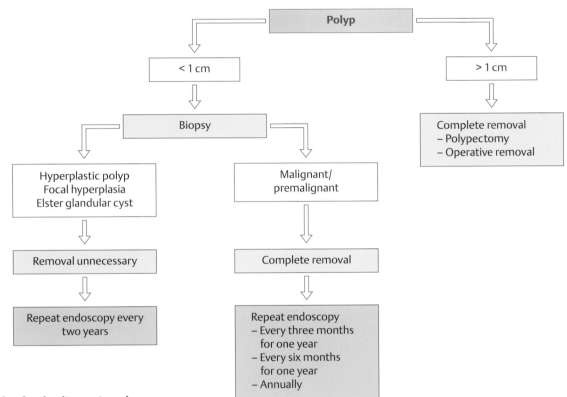

Fig. 3.**104 Algorithm for the diagnosis and treatment of gastric polyps**

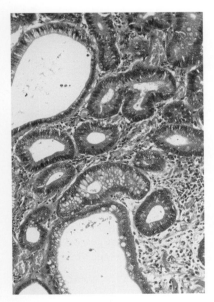
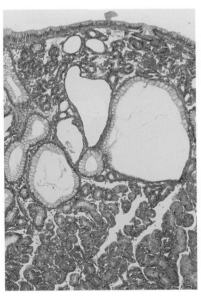
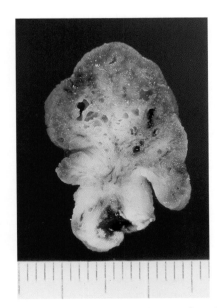

Fig. 3.**105 Histological and pathological features of gastric polyps**

a Histological appearance of tubular adenoma: tubular formations lined with benign neoplastic epithelium

b Histological appearance of a glandular cyst specimen

c Cut surface of a hyperplastic polyp, displaying a typical spongy pattern (all figures from: Hahn and Riemann, *Klinische Gastroenterologie*. Vol. I, 3rd ed. Stuttgart: Thieme 1996)

Malignant Diseases of the Stomach: Gastric Carcinoma, Early Carcinoma

Malignant diseases of the stomach can arise from the epithelium, the lymphatic tissue of the gastric mucosa, and from the connective, supportive, and neurogenic tissues of the stomach wall. Carcinoids and metastases are also found in the stomach (Table 3.**19**).

Table 3.**19** **Malignant gastric tumors and their frequency**

▶ Primary gastric carcinoma	> 80 %
▶ Non-Hodgkin lymphoma	< 5 %
▶ Metastases	< 5 %
▶ Leiomyosarcoma	< 2 %
▶ Carcinoid	< 2 %

■ Gastric Carcinoma

By far the most common malignant tumor of the stomach is gastric carcinoma, usually adenocarcinoma. The histological types are listed in Table 3.**20**.

Role of endoscopy. It is important from a prognostic standpoint to differentiate early gastric carcinoma confined to the mucosa and submucosa from advanced gastric carcinoma that has infiltrated the muscularis propria. It should be noted that the diagnosis of early carcinoma is made postoperatively, not by endoscopic biopsy. The five-year survival rate in patients operated for early gastric cancer is between 70 % and 90 %, as opposed to less than 10 % with advanced gastric carcinoma. This is why the endoscopic diagnosis of early malignant changes is of such major importance. The most reliable method for the early detection of gastric carcinoma is the close follow-up of every ulcerated gastric lesion by endoscopic biopsy. Patients at high risk (Table 3.**21**) should undergo regular endoscopic examinations. Clinical presentation is not a useful parameter in the detection of early malignant changes.

Follow-up intervals. Follow-up intervals of several years are recommended in patients with chronic atrophic gastritis, type B gastritis with lymphocytic infiltration, or intestinal metaplasia.

Table 3.**20** **Malignant epithelial gastric tumors**

▶ Adenocarcinoma
– Papillary
– Tubular
– Mucinous
– Signet-ring cell carcinoma
▶ Adenosquamous carcinoma
▶ Squamous cell carcinoma
▶ Undifferentiated carcinoma

Table 3.**21** **Gastric carcinoma: precancerous conditions and lesions**

▶ Chronic atrophic gastritis (type A gastritis)
▶ H. pylori–associated gastritis (type B gastritis)
▶ Adenomatous gastric polyps
▶ Stomach with hyperplastic polyps
▶ Operated stomach
▶ Positive family history
▶ Ménétrier disease

Intervals of two to three years are appropriate for patients who have undergone partial gastrectomy more than 10 years before, have had hyperplastic polyps removed, or have a positive family history of gastric cancer.

Patients who have Ménétrier disease or have had adenomas removed should be reexamined once a year.

Location. Carcinoma may occur anywhere in the stomach. The most common sites of occurrence are the antrum and lesser curvature, followed by the cardia, fundus, and greater curvature, although the prevalence data vary.

■ Early Carcinoma

Early gastric cancers are classified into three types based on their macroscopic features (Fig. 3.**106**).

▶ Type I, protruding type
  – This type presents mainly as a polypoid lesion. Neither its gross appearance nor its size allow for benign/malignant differentiation.
▶ Type II, superficial type
  – This type is difficult to detect, especially IIb. Endoscopy may show only a subtle difference in color or mucosal appearance relative to the surroundings. The shallow depression in type IIc may be mistaken for an ulcer scar.
▶ Type III, excavating type
  – This type resembles a peptic ulcer at endoscopy, making it the most important lesion requiring differentiation from a benign gastric ulcer.

Because the pathogenesis of the ulcer in early carcinoma is like that of a benign ulcer, the gross and histological findings may fail to identify it as a malignant process. Hence it is important to maintain endoscopic and biopsy surveillance, even during the healing stage of an ulcer.

Fig. 3.**106 Endoscopic classification of early gastric carcinoma**

Mucosa and submucosa
Muscularis propria
Carcinoma
Type I: protruding

a b c
Carcinoma
Type II: superficial, IIa slightly raised, IIb flat, IIc slightly depressed

Carcinoma
Type III: excavating

Malignant Diseases of the Stomach: Advanced Gastric Carcinoma

■ Classification

The morphological forms of advanced gastric carcinoma were classified by Borrmann into four types (Figs. 3.**107**, 3.**108**):

▶ Type I, polypoid form
  – This is a frequently broad-based, polypoid lesion that is virtually indistinguishable from a benign epithelial polyp by its macroscopic features. This type is seen in approximately 30% of cases.
▶ Type II, polypoid form with ulceration
  – The distinguishing endoscopic feature of this carcinoma is its exophytic growth with central ulceration, producing a craterlike appearance. Biopsy specimens should be taken from the margin, as the center is necrotic. This type is also seen in approximately 30% of cases.
▶ Type III, infiltrating form with ulceration
  – Type III is a shallow infiltrating cancer that undermines the mucosa and shows superficial ulceration. This can make it difficult to distinguish from a benign ulcer. It may be poorly demarcated from its surroundings, and the adjacent undermined mucosa frequently appears normal. Biopsy specimens should be taken from the ulcer margin. This type is seen in approximately 10% of cases and tends to metastasize early, implying a very poor prognosis.
▶ Type IV, diffusely infiltrating form
  – The extent of submucosal infiltration by this tumor cannot be determined by endoscopy. The mucosa is irregular, and the stomach wall is firm, indurated, and nondistensible. In some cases the submucosal growth leads to stricture formation. This type, seen in approximately 30% of cases, tends to metastasize early and is usually very extensive when diagnosed.

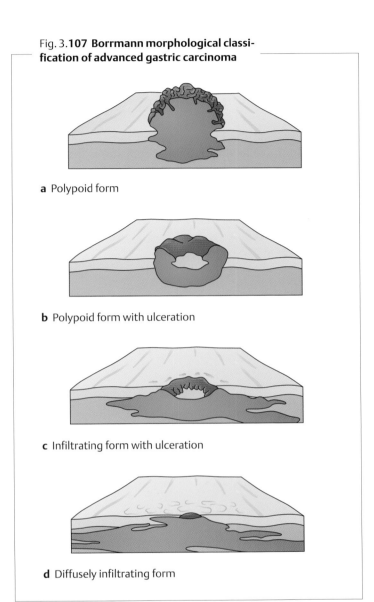

Fig. 3.**107 Borrmann morphological classification of advanced gastric carcinoma**

a Polypoid form

b Polypoid form with ulceration

c Infiltrating form with ulceration

d Diffusely infiltrating form

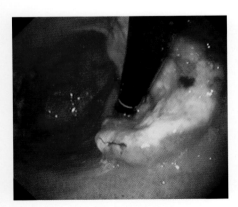

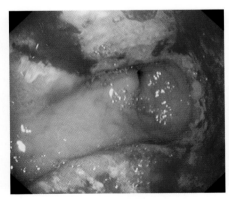

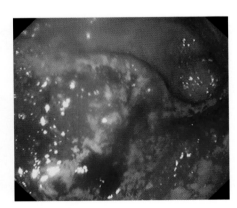

Fig. 3.**108 Advanced gastric carcinoma**
a Tumor in the cardia region. Histology: undifferentiated carcinoma

b Infiltration of surrounding tissues

c Polypoid tumor

Malignant Diseases of the Stomach: Diagnosis of Gastric Carcinoma

■ Diagnosis

 Endoscopic diagnostic criteria

The endoscopic appearance of gastric carcinoma depends on its stage and the primary type of tumor growth (see above). In the following outline of endoscopic features, it should be kept in mind that a tumor cannot be classified as early carcinoma by endoscopic biopsy, but only after it has been surgically removed.

Early carcinoma (Fig. 3.**109**)
▶ Type I, protruding type
  – Polypoid protrusion
  – Mucosa may appear normal, irregular, or erythematous
▶ Type II, superficial type
  – Mucosa discolored, irregular, or nodular
  – IIa: minimally raised
  – IIb: flat
  – IIc: minimally depressed
▶ Type III, excavating type
  – Craterlike excavation
  – Central ulceration

Advanced carcinoma (Fig. 3.**110**)
▶ Type I, polypoid form
  – Broad-based polypoid tumor
  – Mucosa irregular, fissured, or cauliflowerlike
  – Relatively well demarcated from surroundings

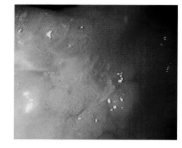

Fig. 3.**109** **Early gastric carcinoma, type IIa**

▶ Type II, polypoid form with ulceration
  – Fungating tumor
  – Central ulceration
  – Craterlike
  – Ulcer base smooth, nodular, or necrotic
  – Relatively well demarcated from surroundings
▶ Type III, infiltrating form with ulceration
  – Superficial ulceration
  – Poorly demarcated from surroundings
  – Shallow undermining of the surrounding mucosa
▶ Type IV, diffusely infiltrating form
  – Mucosa irregular, nodular, or indurated
  – Firm or hard consistency of the stomach wall
  – Stricture formation
  – Altered peristalsis

Differential diagnosis
▶ Benign ulcer
▶ Benign polyp
▶ Gastritis
▶ Lymphoma

Checklist for endoscopic evaluation
▶ Type of growth
▶ Surface characteristics
▶ Consistency
▶ Location
▶ Craniocaudal extent
▶ Relation to surroundings

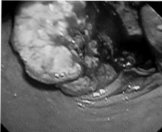 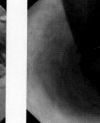

Fig. 3.**110** **Advanced gastric carcinoma**
a Type I
b Type II

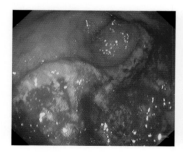 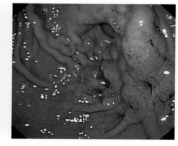

c Type III
d Type IV

Additional Studies
▶ Biopsy
▶ Endosonography
▶ Usual staging work-up: chest radiograph, abdominal ultrasound, abdominal computed tomography (CT), tumor markers for follow-up.

■ Treatment

The treatment of choice is surgical resection. Mucosectomy is an experimental therapy that should be reserved for specialized investigations and centers.

Malignant Diseases of the Stomach: Gastric Lymphoma

■ Clinical Aspects

Gastric lymphoma may be a primary extranodal lesion, or a generalized, primary nodal lymphoma may infiltrate the gastric mucosa secondarily. Primary gastric lymphoma arises from mucosa-associated lymphoid tissue (MALT).

Chronic *H. pylori* infection plays a major role in the pathogenesis of MALT lymphomas. Gastric lymphoma has a considerably better prognosis than gastric carcinoma, with a reported five-year survival rate of 50–90%.

■ Diagnosis

Endoscopic diagnostic criteria (Figs. 3.**111**, 3.**113**)

- No typical features. In some cases the mucosa appears almost normal, in others it appears gastritic with patchy erythema and a bumpy surface.
- Ulcerations: superficial or deep, with or without raised edges, multiple, bizarre
- Polypoid growth is sometimes seen.
- Location: ubiquitous, with a predilection for the gastric body and antrum

Differential diagnosis
- ▶ Gastric carcinoma
- ▶ Gastritis

Checklist for endoscopic evaluation
- ▶ Description of morphological features
- ▶ Location
- ▶ Extent

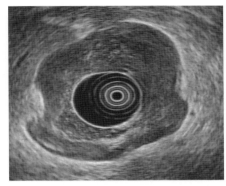

Fig. 3.**112** **Endosonographic image of a high-grade non-Hodgkin lymphoma of the stomach**

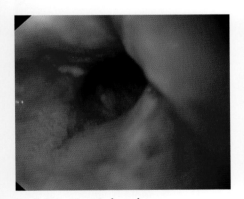

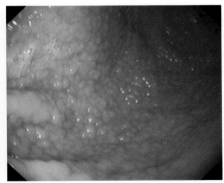

Fig. 3.**111** **Gastric lymphomas**
a High-grade non-Hodgkin lymphoma of the stomach

b MALT lymphoma of the stomach

Additional Studies

To plan treatment that is appropriate for the stage of the disease, it is necessary to localize ("map") the findings in the stomach and look for additional manifestations.
- ▶ Biopsies
  - Eight to ten biopsies from the gross lesion
  - Systematic biopsies from grossly normal-appearing mucosa
    Antrum: four biopsies (one per quadrant)
    Body: four biopsies (one per quadrant)
    Fundus: two biopsies
- ▶ Endosonography (Fig. 3.**112**)
- ▶ Staging work-up
  - Ear, nose, and throat (ENT) examination
  - Differential blood count
  - Bone-marrow aspiration
  - Chest radiograph
  - Thoracic CT

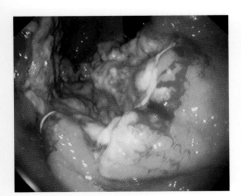

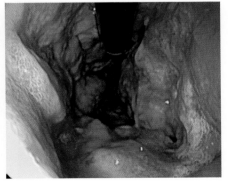

c Ulcerated gastric lymphoma

d MALT lymphoma of the stomach

Malignant Diseases of the Stomach: Gastric Lymphoma, Treatment

■ Stages and Treatment Options

The following treatment options are available for gastric lymphoma:

▶ *H. pylori* eradication
▶ Surgical resection
▶ Irradiation
▶ Chemotherapy

The use of these treatment modalities depends on the tumor grade and the extent of disease (Table 3.**22**).

Table 3.**22**   **Staging of primary gastric lymphomas**

E*	Affected organs and lymph nodes
EI1	Unifocal or multifocal gastric involvement without lymph node involvement and without organ infiltration by contiguous spread. Lymphoma is confined to the mucosa and submucosa.
EI2	Like EI1, but transcending the submucosa and infiltrating the muscularis or serosa or invading an organ by contiguous spread.
EII1	Unifocal or multifocal gastric involvement plus involvement of regional lymph nodes (compartments 1–2).
EII2	Unifocal or multifocal gastric and lymph node involvement going beyond the regional lymph nodes (compartments 1–2) plus further organ involvement by contiguous spread or other localized organ involvement below the diaphragm.
EIII	Unifocal or multifocal gastric or lymph node involvement above or below the diaphragm plus further localized organ involvement, which may be above the diaphragm.
EIV	Unifocal or multifocal gastric involvement with or without involvement of adjacent lymph nodes and diffuse or disseminated involvement of one or more extragastric organs.

* E = primary extranodal disease

Treatment of Low-Grade Non-Hodgkin Lymphoma

▶ *H. pylori* eradication should be considered as a solitary treatment only in patients with low-grade unifocal or multifocal gastric lymphoma without lymph node involvement and without organ infiltration by contiguous spread. This is an organ-conserving strategy, and the response should be regularly assessed by endoscopy. If the treatment is unsuccessful, surgical resection is indicated.
▶ In cases with involvement of regional or nonregional infradiaphragmatic lymph nodes, treatment consists of surgery or irradiation.
▶ With extensive spread (infradiaphragmatic and supradiaphragmatic lymph nodes, involvement of additional organs), chemotherapy is indicated.

Treatment of High-Grade Non-Hodgkin Lymphoma

▶ High-grade non-Hodgkin lymphoma is an indication for chemotherapy, which may be combined with surgical resection (early stage) or irradiation (early and advanced stages).

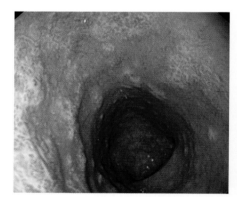

Fig. 3.**113 a–d**   **MALT lymphomas of the stomach**

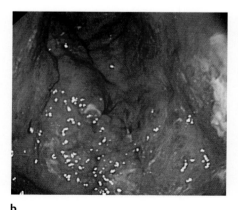

b

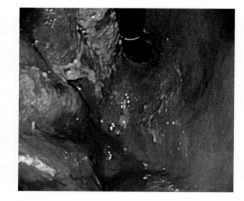

c

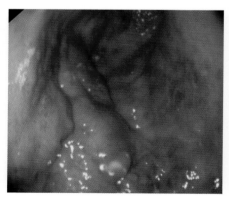

d

Portal Hypertension and Hypertensive Gastropathy: Clinical Aspects

■ Causes and Findings

Hypertensive gastropathy (Fig. 3.**114**). Hypertensive gastropathy is seen in patients with portal hypertension. While histology shows scant inflammatory mucosal infiltrate, the gastric mucosa exhibits significant epithelial or vascular damage. Given the nondescript histological changes, the diagnosis is based primarily on endoscopic findings.

Gastric antral venous ectasia (GAVE) syndrome (Fig. 3.**115**). GAVE syndrome refers to the ectatic dilatation of venous plexuses in the gastric antrum due to portal hypertension (synonym: "watermelon stomach"). Oozing hemorrhages are not uncommon.

Varices (Fig. 3.**116**). Patients with portal hypertension sometimes develop varices in the gastric fundus and cardia, which accompany the esophageal varices. Isolated gastric varices are sometimes found in association with splenic vein thrombosis, which is usually secondary to a tumor or pancreatitis. In rare cases, veins showing varixlike dilatation may extend into the gastric body, antrum, and duodenum.

■ Treatment

Prophylactic endoscopic treatment is not recommended. Bleeding varices in the fundus and cardia are discussed on page 150.

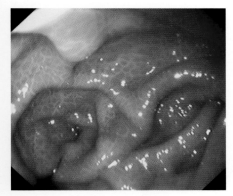

Fig. 3.**114 a–d** **Hypertensive gastropathy.** Pronounced snakeskin-like pattern of mucosal markings

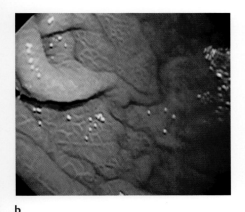

b

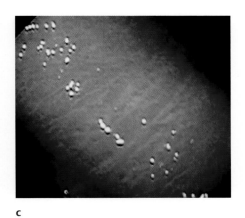

c

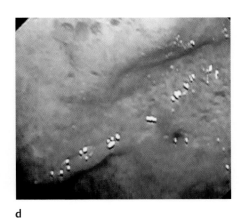

d

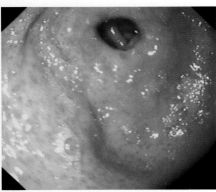
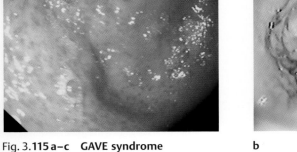

Fig. 3.**115 a–c** **GAVE syndrome**

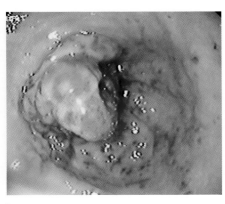

b

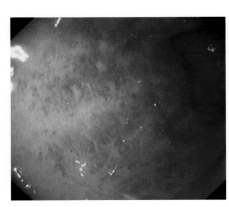

c

Portal Hypertension and Hypertensive Gastropathy: Diagnosis

 Endoscopic diagnostic criteria

▶ Hypertensive gastropathy (Fig. 3.**114**)
- – Stippled erythema
- – Edema
- – Snake-skin pattern of mucosal markings
- – Confluent areas of erythema
- – Superficial hemorrhages
▶ GAVE syndrome (Fig. 3.**115**)
- – Patchy, streaky, or reticular pattern of erythema
- – Mucosal hemorrhages
- – Streaks radiating toward the antrum ("watermelon stripes")
- – Fragile mucosa
▶ Varices (Fig. 3.**116**)
- – Convoluted vessels protruding into the lumen, sometimes with a "cluster of grapes" appearance; mucosa over the varices may be normal, dull red, or bluish
- – Encircling the cardia or fundus; sometimes found in the body and antrum, rarely in the duodenum

Differential diagnosis

▶ Varices/mucosal folds
▶ Hypertensive gastropathy/gastritis

Checklist for endoscopic evaluation

▶ Determine location of varices in the stomach.
▶ Estimate severity.
▶ Look for varices in the esophagus.
▶ Check for signs of hypertensive gastropathy.

Additional Studies

▶ If in doubt, endosonography can differentiate between a varix and a thick fold of mucosa (Fig. 3.**117**).

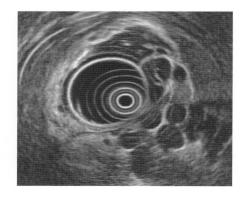

Fig. 3.**117 Endosonography of gastric varices**

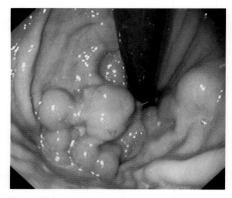

Fig. 3.**116 Gastric varices**
a Fundic varices

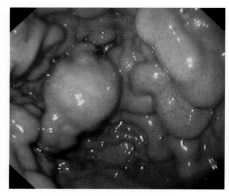

b, c Body and fundic varices secondary to splenic vein thrombosis

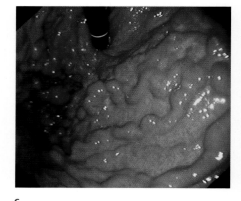

c

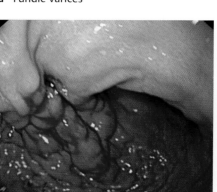

d Varicose venous dilatation in the stomach due to portal hypertension, with signs of fresh hemorrhage

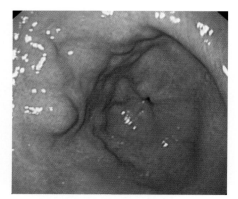

e Prepyloric varicose gastric veins

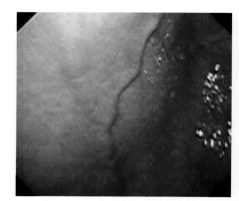

f Antral varix due to portal vein thrombosis in a patient with pancreatic carcinoma

The Operated Stomach

■ Special Considerations

The operated stomach is a challenge for the endoscopist in two respects: First, anatomical orientation is difficult and often the stomach is difficult to examine. Second, different types of resections are associated with different complications, some of which are detectable by endoscopy. It is important for the examiner to know the prior history, therefore (Tables 3.**23**, 3.**24**).

Table 3.**23** **Information needed before examining the operated stomach**

> ▶ Reason for the operation: benign/malignant disease
> ▶ Date of the operation
> ▶ Type of resection performed

Table 3.**24** **Types of surgery most commonly seen by endoscopists**

> ▶ Total gastrectomy
> ▶ Partial gastrectomy
> ▶ Vagotomy with or without pyloroplasty
> ▶ Fundoplication

■ Systematic Examination

As in the nonoperated stomach, endoscopy of the postsurgical stomach should follow a systematic routine. The gastroesophageal junction, gastric remnant, anastomosis, and afferent and efferent loops are inspected, and the fundus and cardia are examined in retroflexion (Fig. 3.**118**).

Complications that arise in association with gastric operations can be classified as early (perioperative) or late (Table 3.**25**).

Table 3.**25** **Complications following gastric surgery**

Early complications
▶ Detectable by endoscopy
– Hemorrhage
– Anastomotic stenosis
▶ Not detectable by endoscopy
– Gastric atony
– Anastomotic leak

Late complications
▶ Detectable by endoscopy
– Recurrence of the underlying disease: carcinoma, ulcer
– Obstruction: postoperative stenosis, stricture due to ulcer scarring, occasional efferent loop syndrome
– Bezoars
– Suture remnants
– Reflux-induced complications: alkaline reflux esophagitis, alkaline reflux gastropathy
– Anastomotic ulcer
– Anastomositis
– Gastric remnant carcinoma
▶ Not detectable by endoscopy
– Dumping syndrome (early and late)
– Metabolic deficiency states: iron deficiency, calcium deficiency, vitamin B_{12} deficiency, vitamin D deficiency

Fig. 3.**118a–f Systematic examination of the operated stomach**

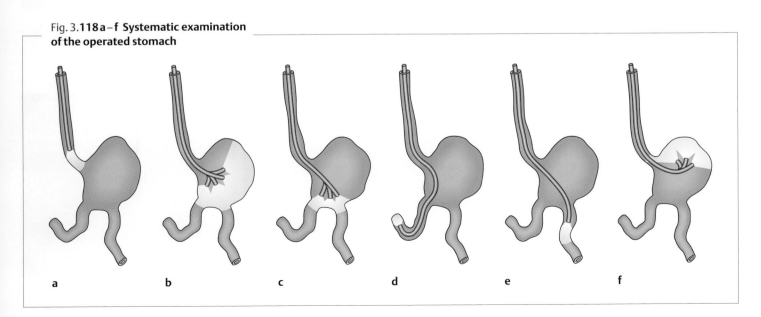

a   b   c   d   e   f

The Operated Stomach: Endoscopically Identifiable Lesions and Diseases

■ Alkaline Reflux Gastropathy

It is very common to find erythematous and sometimes bile-tinged mucosa just proximal to the stoma in the operated stomach. Histologically, inflammatory mucosal changes are found in 60–90 % of cases. It is likely that the reflux of bile and alkaline pancreatic juice has causal significance. The degree of macroscopic and histological changes does not correlate with the severity of the complaints, and many patients are asymptomatic. The endoscopic picture is characterized by edema, erythema, and mucosal fragility when biliary secretions are present.

■ Reflux Esophagitis

Inflammatory changes in the distal esophagus are particularly common after total gastrectomy but may also be seen after partial gastrectomy, especially in cases with stenotic or functional obstruction of the efferent loop (Fig. 3.**119 a**).

■ Stenoses

Anastomotic stenoses may result from a primary tight stoma or from recurrent ulceration with cicatricial stricturing. Stenoses are often difficult to identify endoscopically, and an upper gastrointestinal contrast series should be obtained in doubtful cases.

■ Ulcers

Ulcerations may develop after vagotomy as a recurrence of the underlying disease or may occur close to the stoma following partial gastrectomy (Fig. 3.**119 b**). They are usually found just beyond the stoma but occasionally occur proximal to it. Possible causes are residual antrum remaining in the stomach, an antral remnant at the duodenal stump, Zollinger–Ellison syndrome, hyperparathyroidism, a tight stoma, or ischemia.

■ Suture Granuloma

In rare cases, suture material may be found at the site of the anastomosis (Fig. 3.**119 c**). This can lead to chronic occult blood loss.

■ Bezoars

Bezoars are rounded, compressed aggregations of fruit and vegetable fibers (Fig. 3.**119 d**). They may be seen following vagotomy and partial resections. They probably result from a motility disorder, and a narrow gastric outlet may be contributory. Large bezoars can cause obstructive symptoms.

■ Gastric Remnant Carcinoma

Gastric remnant carcinomas occur from 10–15 years after a partial gastrectomy. Endoscopy may show erosions, ulcerations, mucosal fragility, or a polypoid lesion. Early diagnosis can be difficult. For this reason, generous biopsy specimens should be taken from around the stoma even when subtle mucosal changes are found. Carcinomas can occur anywhere in the gastric remnant, even at multiple sites.

■ Recurrent Carcinoma

Whereas gastric remnant carcinoma develops after a prolonged interval, recurrent cancer generally occurs within a few years after surgery for gastric carcinoma. Consequently, it is recommended that endoscopic follow-ups be scheduled at intervals from three months to one year after the primary operation.

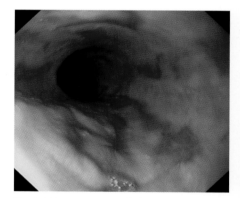

Fig. 3.**119   Lesions and diseases in the operated stomach**
a   Inflammatory changes in the distal esophagus following gastrectomy

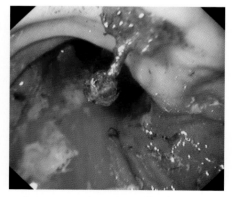

b   Anastomotic ulcer following a Billroth II gastroenterostomy

c   Suture granuloma in a Billroth II stomach

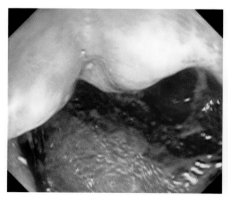

d   Bezoar

Total Gastrectomy

When the entire stomach is removed, the stump of the esophagus is anastomosed to the small intestine. This may take the form of an end-to-end anastomosis (Fig. 3.**120a**) or end-to-side anastomosis (Fig. 3.**120b**), or a substitute gastric reservoir may be constructed (Fig. 3.**120c**).

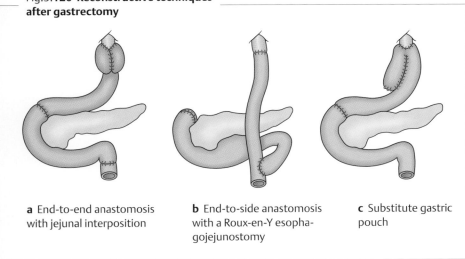

Fig.3.**120 Reconstructive techniques after gastrectomy**

a End-to-end anastomosis with jejunal interposition

b End-to-side anastomosis with a Roux-en-Y esophagojejunostomy

c Substitute gastric pouch

 Normal findings (Figs. 3.**121 a, b**)

▶ The anastomosis is located at 35–40 cm.
▶ Grayish, small bowel mucosa, differing from the reddish–yellow gastric mucosa, is seen proximal to the ring.
▶ Usually the endoscope can be advanced another 35–40 cm.
▶ Two lumina separated by a cardialike ridge are sometimes seen (depending on the surgical technique).

Checklist for endoscopic evaluation

▶ Inspect the esophagus for inflammatory changes.
▶ Locate the anastomosis.
▶ Check distance from the incisor teeth in centimeters.
▶ For primary malignant disease: evidence of recurrence?

Pathological findings (Fig. 3.**121 c**)

▶ Erosions proximal to the anastomosis
▶ Anastomotic ulcer
▶ Anastomositis
▶ Recurrent carcinoma

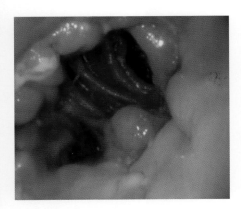
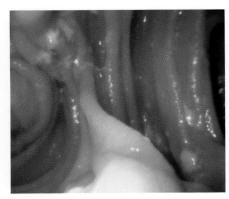
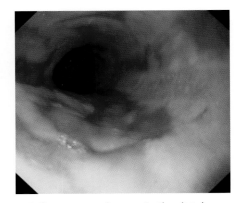

Fig. 3.**121 Gastrectomy**
a View of the anastomosis

b End-to-side anastomosis

c Inflammatory changes in the distal esophagus

Partial Gastrectomy: Types and Findings

■ Types

The most common types of partial gastrectomy are the Billroth I operation (hemigastrectomy with gastroduodenostomy; Fig. 3.**122 a**), the Billroth II operation (hemigastrectomy with gastrojejunostomy; Fig. 3.**122 b**), with or without a Braun side-to-side anastomosis (Fig. 3.**122 c**), and the Roux-en-Y gastrojejunostomy (Fig. 3.**122 d**).

Billroth I. The Billroth I stomach can usually be examined endoscopically without difficulties. This is also true of a Roux-en-Y gastrojejunostomy, although the Y anastomosis usually cannot be inspected as it may be up to 50 cm distal to the gastrojejunostomy.

Billroth II. Examination of the Billroth II stomach is not always easy, as the afferent loop should be inspected as far as the stump, while the efferent loop should be inspected as far distally as possible. The Braun side-to-side anastomosis cannot always be visualized.

■ Endoscopic Appearance

 Normal findings

▶ A large range of normal findings are seen at the anastomotic ring, which may appear flat, raised, or nodular.
▶ The extent of the resection and course of the anastomosis are also highly variable.
▶ Billroth I stomach (Fig. 3.**123 a**)
  – Mucosal folds end abruptly at the stoma
  – The stoma may have a nodular appearance
  – The mucosa may appear normal
  – Lesser curvature is usually deformed and sometimes creased
▶ Billroth II stomach (Fig. 3.**123 b**)
  – Highly variable
  – Efferent loop is usually easier to intubate, generally lying in direct continuity with the gastric lumen
  – Afferent loop is usually more difficult to intubate, terminates in a blind pouch; biliary secretions are found
  – Anastomotic ring is highly variable in appearance
▶ Roux-en-Y gastrojejunostomy
  – Only one loop can be intubated
  – Anastomosis of the afferent loop is up to 50 cm past the gastrojejunostomy, so usually it cannot be identified
  – No evidence of biliary secretions in the stomach
  – Little erythema at the anastomosis

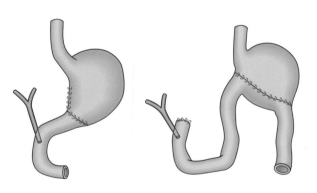

Fig. 3.**122 Reconstructive techniques after partial gastrectomy**

a Billroth I operation (partial gastrectomy with gastroduodenostomy)

b Billroth II operation (partial gastrectomy with gastrojejunostomy)

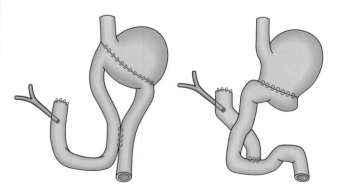

c Billroth II operation with a Braun side-to-side anastomosis

d Billroth II operation with a Roux-en-Y gastro-jejunostomy

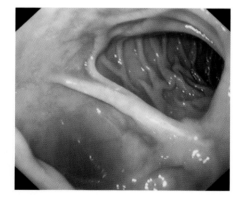

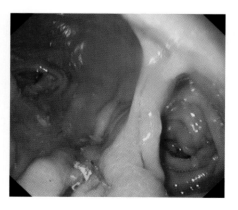

Fig. 3.**123 Normal findings after partial gastrectomy**
a Billroth I operation. View of the anastomosis

b Billroth II operation. View of the anastomosis, with afferent and efferent loops

Partial Gastrectomy: Examination

Checklist for endoscopic evaluation
- Inspect the esophagus, particularly the gastroesophageal junction.
- Inspect the gastric remnant.
- Inspect the anastomotic ring.
- Billroth I stomach and Roux-en-Y gastrojejunostomy
  - Inspect the efferent loop.
- Billroth II stomach (Fig. 3.**124**)
  - Inspect the afferent loop as far as the stump.
  - Inspect the efferent loop as far as the Braun anastomosis, if present.

Pathological findings (Fig. 3.**125**)
- Reflux esophagitis
- Redness, erythema, erosion at the anastomotic site
- Increased fragility of the mucosa
- Nodule formation at the anastomosis
- Polypoid mucosa
- Ulcerations
- Neoplastic, carcinomatous mucosal changes
- Anastomotic stenosis
- Bezoar in the gastric remnant
- Biliary secretion in the gastric remnant

Additional Studies
- Generous biopsy
- Upper gastrointestinal series

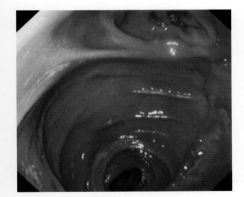

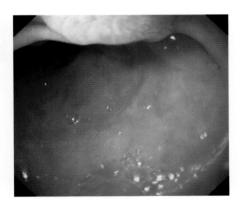

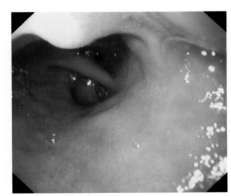

Fig. 3.**124** **Billroth II operation**
a View of the afferent and efferent loops

b View of the major papilla

c The endoscope has been advanced into the afferent loop

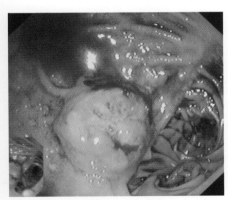

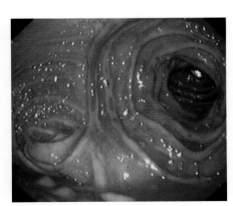

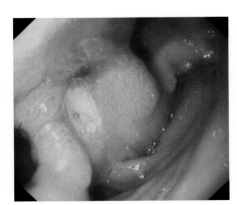

Fig. 3.**125** **Pathological findings after partial gastrectomy**
a Carcinoma in the operated stomach (Billroth II)

b Mild mucosal erythema at the Braun anastomosis

c Gastroenterostomy with an ulcer at the anastomotic site

Vagotomy and Fundoplication

■ Vagotomy and Pyloroplasty

Vagotomy (truncal vagotomy and selective proximal vagotomy), with or without a Heineke–Mikulicz pyloroplasty, is rarely performed today. The endoscopist is still occasionally confronted with these postoperative states, however. In the Heineke–Mikulicz pyloroplasty, the gastric outlet is incised longitudinally and reapproximated transversely (Fig. 3.**126**). This produces a semicircular fold in the duodenal bulb, with a typical endoscopic appearance.

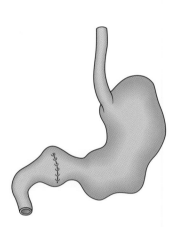

Fig. 3.**126 Heineke–Mikulicz pyloroplasty.** The gastric outlet is incised longitudinally and reapproximated transversely

■ Fundoplication

In the classic fundoplication, the fundus is wrapped around the juxtacardial esophagus and secured with sutures, thereby narrowing the cardia and creating an acute angle at the gastric inlet (Fig. 3.**127 a**). Fundoplication has been and is practiced in a modified form for reflux esophagitis that is refractory to medical therapy.

Fig. 3.**127 Fundoplication**

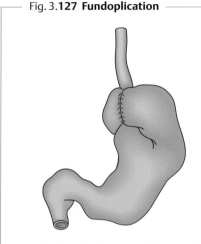
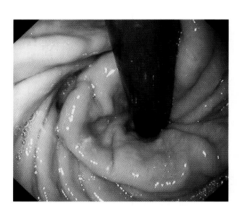

a The fundus is wrapped like a cuff around the juxtacardial esophagus and secured with sutures

b Retroflexed view of a plicated fundus

■ Endoscopic Appearance

Typical findings

▶ After vagotomy alone
  – Usually no particular findings
▶ After truncal vagotomy
  – Increased incidence of bezoars
▶ Vagotomy with pyloroplasty
  – Gaping pylorus
  – Semicircular fold caused by the opened pylorus

Checklist for endoscopic evaluation

▶ Inspect the enlarged pylorus

Pathological findings

▶ Mucosal erythema in the proximal pylorus
▶ Erosions
▶ Ulcerations
▶ Bezoars

■ Endoscopic Appearance

Typical findings (Fig. 3.127 b)

▶ Deformation of the cardia
▶ Thickened cardial ring
▶ Soft, symmetrical mucosal ring

Differential diagnosis

▶ Submucosal tumor in the cardia region

Checklist for endoscopic evaluation

▶ Evaluate gastroesophageal junction.
▶ Check resistance to endoscope passage.
▶ Evaluate cardial closure with the retroflexed scope.

Pathological findings

▶ Recurrence of reflux esophagitis
▶ Cardial closure too tight

Angiodysplasias

■ Definition

Angiodysplasia is a collective term for a heterogeneous group of vascular abnormalities in the gastric mucosa. Angiodysplasias are seen in the absence of a detectable underlying disease, in the setting of hereditary disorders (Osler disease, von Willebrandt–Jürgen syndrome), and in acquired diseases (chronic renal failure, hepatic cirrhosis, irradiation, connective tissue diseases).

■ Diagnosis

Angiodysplasias appear endoscopically as bright red spots, flat or raised, ranging from a few millimeters to 1 cm in diameter and occasionally larger. They may be solitary, multiple, or numerous and are a source of chronic oozing hemorrhages leading to iron deficiency (Fig. 3.**128**).

Differentiation is required from suction artifacts, petechial hemorrhages, erosions, and Kaposi sarcoma (Fig. 3.**129**).

A special form is watermelon stomach (GAVE syndrome) occurring in patients with portal hypertension (see p. 119; Fig. 3.**130**).

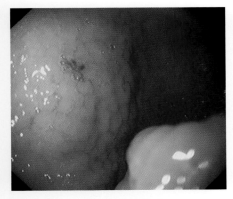
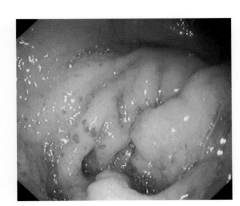
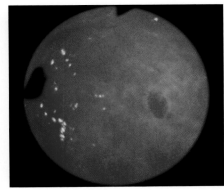

Fig. 3.**128 a–c**   Angiodysplasia

b

c

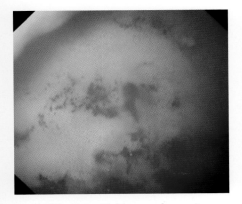
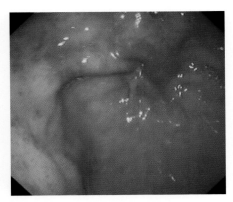
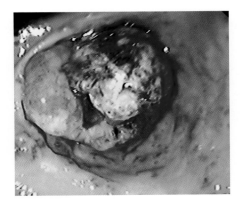

Fig. 3.**129**   **Petechial hemorrhages in thrombocytopenia**

Fig. 3.**130 a, b**   **GAVE syndrome in portal hypertension**

b

Diverticula, Abnormal Gastric Contents

■ Diverticula

Gastric diverticula are uncommon. Most are subcardial, and a smaller percentage are found in the antrum; other sites are rare. Very rare but possible complications are ulceration and hemorrhage. The diagnosis is usually incidental.

Endoscopy demonstrates a round or oval orifice, occasionally with a projecting fold (Fig. 3.**131**).

■ Abnormal Gastric Contents

Gastroscopy will occasionally reveal coatings on the gastric mucosa that are initially difficult to identify. Frequently they consist of drug or food residues (Fig. 3.**132**). Food residues are found in patients who have not been adequately prepared for endoscopy. They are also seen in association with motility disorders and, of course, obstructions.

When endoscopy is performed late in the day, considerably more resting juice is found than in the morning. Bile reflux from the pylorus is sometimes seen, generally as an incidental finding (Fig. 3.**132 e**).

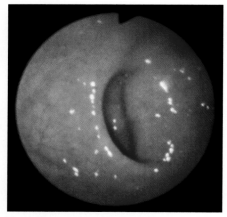

Fig. 3.**131**　**Gastric diverticulum**

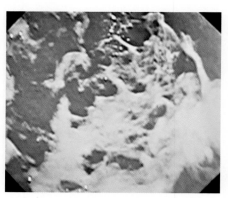

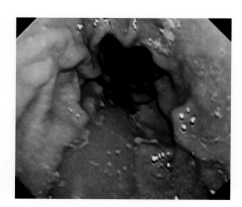

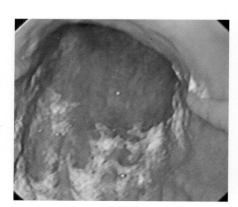

Fig. 3.**132**　**Drug and food residues, bile**
a　Maalox residues

b–d　Gastric juice and food residues

c

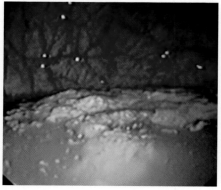

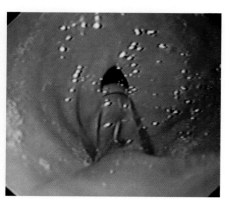

d

e　Bile reflux

Miscellaneous

This section concludes with a review of several interesting findings in the stomach, some of which are not commonly seen (Fig. 3.**133**).

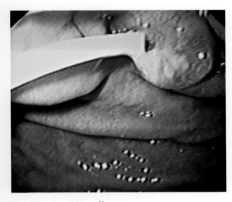

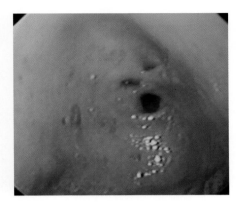

Fig. 3.**133** **Miscellaneous**
a Pancreatic pseudocyst. A drain has perforated into the stomach

b Fistula formation in the pyloric region

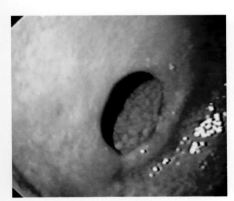

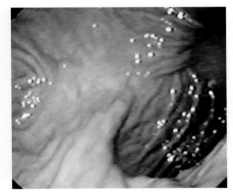

c Pressure injury to the pyloric region from a feeding tube

d Bizarre appearance in a cascade stomach

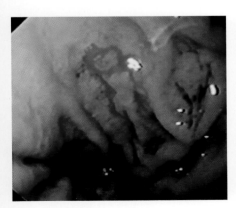

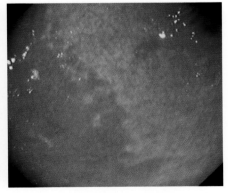

e Suction artifacts

f Sharply demarcated area of intestinal metaplasia

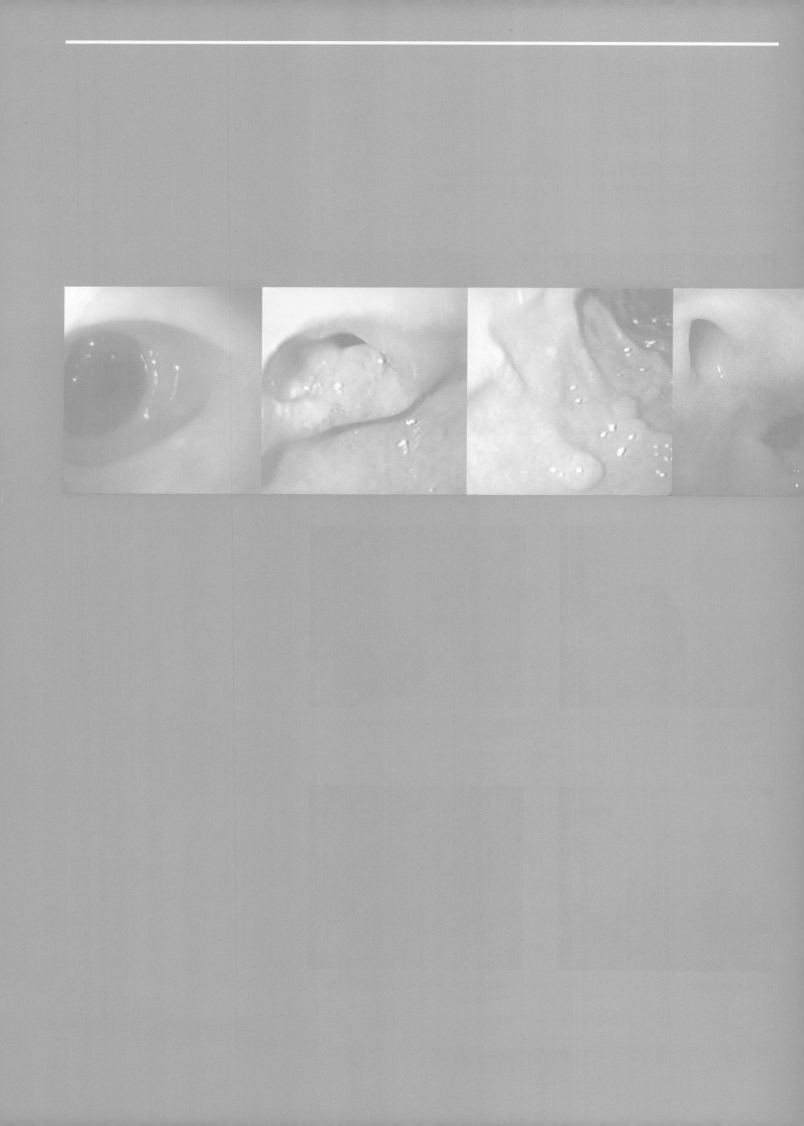

3.3 Pathological Findings: Duodenum

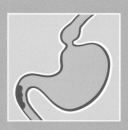

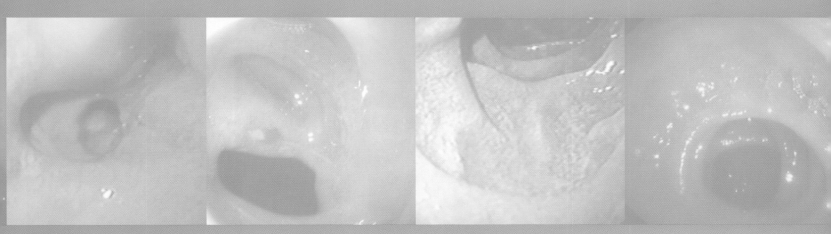

Overview of Pathological Findings in the Duodenum

Table 2.**26** **Pathological findings in the duodenum**

▶ Duodenal ulcer
▶ Bulbitis
▶ Polypoid lesions
▶ Sprue
▶ Crohn disease
▶ Whipple disease
▶ Diverticula
▶ Changes associated with diseases in adjacent organs

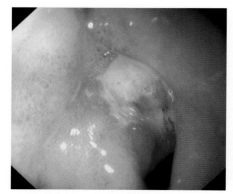

Fig. 3.**134**   Duodenal ulcer

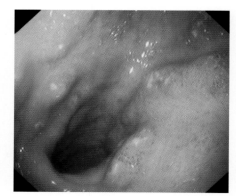

Fig. 3.**135**   Bulbitis

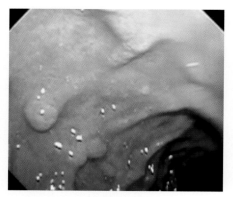

Fig. 3.**136**   Polypoid lesions in the duodenal bulb

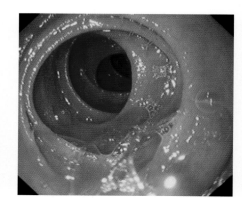

Fig. 3.**137**   Sprue

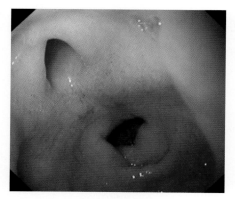

Fig. 3.**138**   Bulbar diverticulum

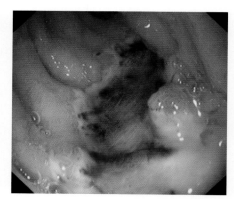

Fig. 3.**139**   Inflammation and necrosis in the duodenum of a patient with pancreatitis

Duodenal Ulcer: Clinical Features

■ Definition and Causes

Duodenal ulcer is an epithelial defect in the bulbar or descending duodenum that penetrates the muscularis mucosae and extends into the submucosa (Fig. 3.**141**). The precipitating causes include *Helicobacter pylori* infection (detectable in more than 90% of cases) and the ingestion of nonsteroidal anti-inflammatory drugs (NSAIDs). Additional risk factors include nicotine abuse, alcohol abuse, and stress.

■ Clinical Aspects

A duodenal ulcer cannot be diagnosed from the clinical presentation alone. The symptoms range from typical nocturnal pain and vague or crampy abdominal discomfort to an almost complete absence of complaints, particularly with NSAID-induced ulcers.

■ Location

Ninety percent of duodenal ulcers occur in the duodenal bulb. Ulcers are usually located on the anterior wall of the bulb, less commonly on the posterior wall and lesser curvature. Ulcers on the greater curvature are rare (Fig. 3.**140**). Multiple "kissing" ulcers are found on the anterior and posterior walls in 10–20% of cases. Ulcers located distal to the bulb should raise suspicion of Zollinger–Ellison syndrome.

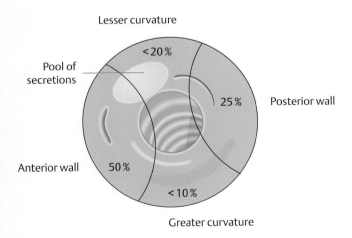

Fig. 3.**140 Frequency distribution of duodenal ulcers**

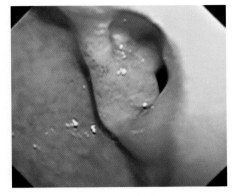

Fig. 3.**141 a–d**   Duodenal ulcer

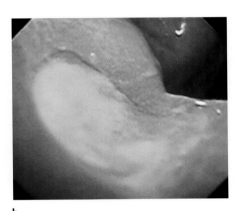

b

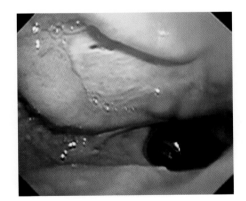

c

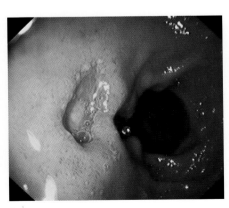

d

Duodenal Ulcer: Diagnosis and Treatment

■ Diagnosis

 Endoscopic diagnostic criteria (Figs. 3.**141**, 3.**142**)

▶ The endoscopic appearance depends on the ulcer stage. Three stages are distinguished: the active stage, healing stage, and scar stage.
▶ Active stage
  – Usually round or oval
  – Oblong, streaklike, linear, irregular
  – Multiple lesions, stippled pattern
  – Usually < 1 cm, but may be larger
  – Inflamed ulcer margin
  – Ulcer base: fibrin-coated, greenish
  – Hematin
  – Visible vessel
▶ Healing stage
  – Flatter ulcer margin
  – Hyperemic mucosa growing from edges to center
  – Reddish mucosa covering the ulcer base
▶ Scar stage
  – Healed epithelial defect
  – Occasional deep niche, deformity due to scarring

Differential diagnosis
▶ Very typical appearance
▶ Very rare: penetrating pancreatic carcinoma
▶ Carcinoid
▶ Crohn disease
▶ Malignant lymphoma
▶ Duodenal carcinoma

Checklist for endoscopic evaluation
▶ Location
  – Duodenal bulb, postbulbar duodenum, anterior or posterior wall of bulb, lesser or greater curvature
  – **Caution:** The posterior wall of the bulb is difficult to inspect. Posterior wall ulcers are easily missed on cursory inspection because they are located on the right, convex side of the curved duodenal bulb in the endoscopic image, and it is easy to look past them.
▶ Size
▶ Number
▶ Shape: round, oval, oblong, linear, bizarre
▶ Ulcer margin
▶ Ulcer base: fresh blood, hematin, fibrin, visible vessel
▶ Assess need for endoscopic treatment.
  – Stages I–IIa should be treated (see p. 151).
  – **Caution:** A bleeding posterior wall ulcer (that has eroded the pancreaticoduodenal artery) requires immediate operative treatment!

Additional Studies
▶ Always biopsy the gastric antrum and body (*H. pylori*?) for histology, rapid urease testing, or both.
▶ Biopsy the ulcer only if it does not heal or in order to exclude a particular diagnosis (Crohn disease).

■ Treatment and Follow-Up

The patient is treated with proton pump inhibitors (PPI). If *H. pylori* is detected, eradication therapy is indicated (see p. 103).

An uncomplicated duodenal ulcer that shows good clinical response does not require endoscopic follow-up. If complaints persist, the patient should undergo repeat endoscopy with biopsy (Crohn disease?), and further tests should be performed to exclude Zollinger–Ellison syndrome.

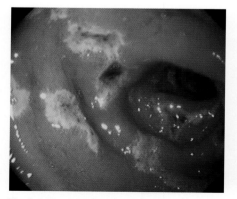
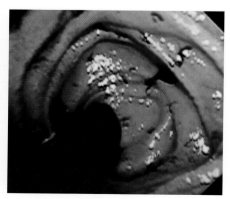
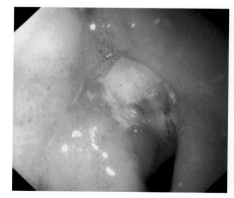

Fig. 3.142 Duodenal ulcer
a Fibrin-coated duodenal ulcer with traces of hematin in an aspirin user

b Traces of hematin

c Rounded ulcer with fibrin coating

Duodenal Ulcer: Complications

■ Bleeding, Penetration, and Perforation

Posterior wall ulcers can result in massive bleeding due to erosion of the adjacent pancreaticoduodenal artery (Figs. 3.**143**, 3.**144**). They may also penetrate into the pancreas. The main complication of anterior wall ulcers is perforation.

Duodenal ulcers are more likely than gastric ulcers to cause wall deformity due to scarring. This can lead to pseudodiverticula and strictures, especially with recurrent ulcers.

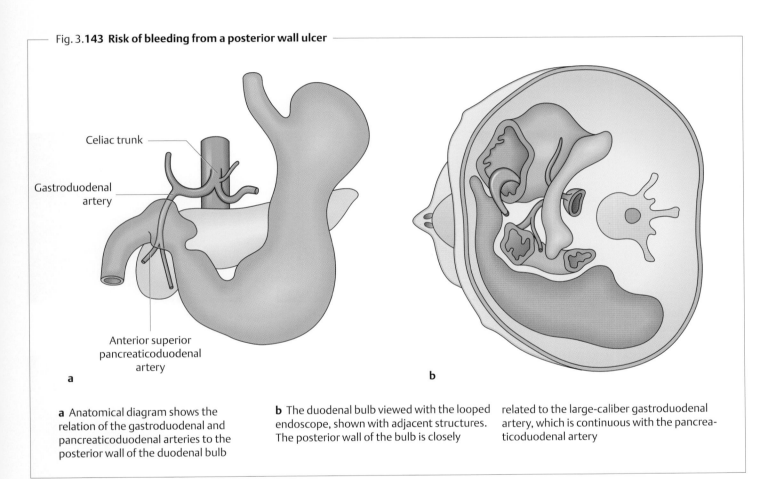

Fig. 3.**143 Risk of bleeding from a posterior wall ulcer**

Celiac trunk

Gastroduodenal artery

Anterior superior pancreaticoduodenal artery

a

b

a Anatomical diagram shows the relation of the gastroduodenal and pancreaticoduodenal arteries to the posterior wall of the duodenal bulb

b The duodenal bulb viewed with the looped endoscope, shown with adjacent structures. The posterior wall of the bulb is closely related to the large-caliber gastroduodenal artery, which is continuous with the pancreaticoduodenal artery

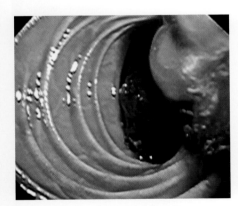

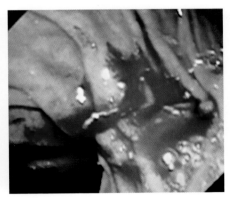

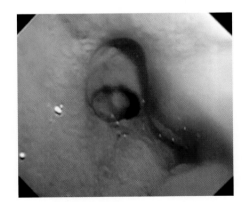

Fig. 3.**144 a, b   Fresh bleeding from a duodenal ulcer**

b

Fig. 3.**145   Duodenal ulcer with perforation**

3

Bulbitis

■ Cause

Peptic duodenitis is believed to result from gastric metaplasia of the duodenal mucosa with subsequent *H. pylori* infection.

■ Diagnosis

 Endoscopic diagnostic criteria (Fig. 3.**146**)

- ▶ Erythema
- ▶ Edema
- ▶ Boggy swelling
- ▶ Erosion: flat, raised
- ▶ Lesions: stippled, spotty, diffuse, patchy, ubiquitous

Differential diagnosis

- ▶ Granular mucosa as a normal variant (Fig. 3.**147**)
- ▶ Heterotopic gastric mucosa
- ▶ Infection (*Salmonella*, *Shigella*)
- ▶ Crohn disease
- ▶ Whipple disease

Checklist for endoscopic evaluation

- ▶ Morphology of the lesions
- ▶ Extent of the lesions

Additional Studies

- ▶ Biopsy

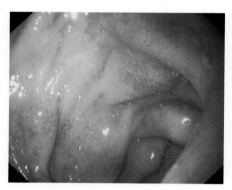

Fig. 3.146 Bulbitis
a Erythematous mucosa

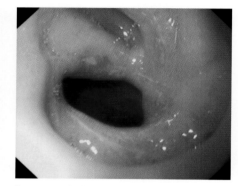

b Erosive bulbitis

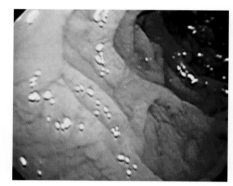

c Edematous bulb

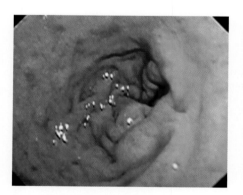

d, e Stippled to spotty lesions

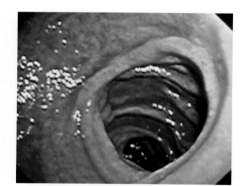

e

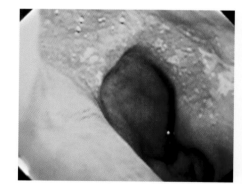

f Ulcerative bulbitis

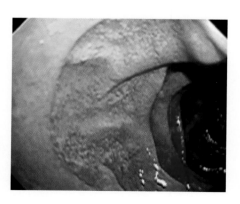

Fig. 3.**147** **Granular mucosa in the duodenal bulb**

Polypoid Lesions in the Duodenum

Polypoid lesions in the duodenum are rare. Their endoscopic appearance may be quite typical (e.g., adenomas), but in doubtful cases the diagnosis is established histologically.

■ Classification

Polypoid lesions can result from inflammatory hyperplasia (most frequent cause), heterotopic tissues (gastric, occasionally pancreatic), lymphofollicular hyperplasia, and Brunner gland hyperplasia. Malignant polyps are very rare. The various types, including rare causes, are summarized in Table 3.27.

Table 3.**27** **Polypoid lesions in the duodenum**

Benign polypoid lesions in the duodenum
► Inflammatory hyperplastic polyps
► Heterotopic gastric mucosa
► Heterotopic pancreatic tissue
► Lymphatic hyperplasia
► Brunner gland hyperplasia
► Mesenchymal tumors (leiomyoma, lipoma)
► Adenoma

Malignant polypoid lesions in the duodenum
► Adenocarcinoma
► Carcinoid
► Lymphoma (Fig. 3.**148 f**)
► Metastases

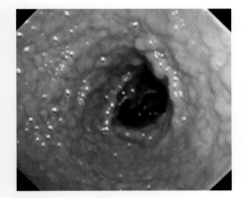

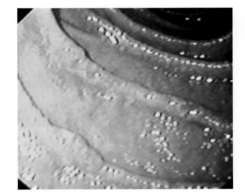

Fig. 3.**148** **Polypoid lesions in the duodenum**
a Heterotopic gastric mucosa

b Heterotopic gastric epithelium

c Ectopic gastric tissue

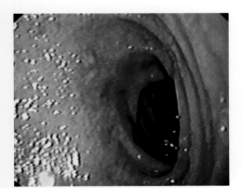

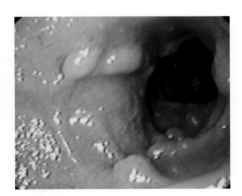

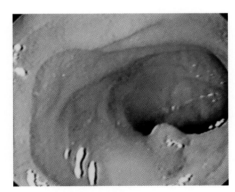

d Polypous mucosa showing coarse granularity

e Boggy, edematous mucosa. Histology showed mild inflammation

f Mucosa-associated lymphoid tissue (MALT) lymphoma in the duodenal bulb

Polypoid Lesions in the Duodenum: Diagnosis

 Checklist for endoscopic evaluation

▶ Location: duodenal bulb, postbulbar duodenum, papilla
▶ Size
▶ Number
▶ Morphology: pedunculated or sessile, mucosal surface

Endoscopic diagnostic criteria for individual polypoid lesions

▶ **Inflammatory hyperplastic polyps** (Figs. 3.**148**, 3.**149**)
  – Most common polypoid lesions in the duodenum
  – Occur in the bulbar and postbulbar duodenum
  – Rarely solitary, usually multiple
  – Small (2–6 mm)
  – Mucosa: unchanged or may be erythematous, eroded, or ulcerated
  – Histology: often shows normal duodenal mucosa
▶ **Heterotopic gastric mucosa** (Fig. 3.**148 a–c**)
  – Found mainly in the postpyloric or postbulbar duodenum
  – Usually multiple, arranged in clusters, or sheetlike
  – Small (2–6 mm)
  – Raised, poorly demarcated from surroundings
  – Mucosa: nodular, erythematous
  – Histology: gastric mucosa, often positive for *H. pylori*

▶ **Brunner gland hyperplasia** (Fig. 3.**148 d**)
  – Occurs throughout the proximal duodenum, including the bulb
  – Usually multiple
  – Small (2–6 mm)
  – Mucosa may be erythematous
▶ **Lymphatic hyperplasia**
  – Found in the second part of the duodenum
  – Usually multiple, arranged in clusters
  – Small (several millimeters)
▶ **Adenomas**
  – Rare
  – Occur in the first and second parts of the duodenum
  – Papilla
  – Solitary or multiple
  – Usually relatively large (> 1 cm)
  – Pedunculated or sessile
  – Mucosa: nodular, eroded, ulcerated
▶ **Leiomyoma**
  – Found mainly between the first and second parts of the duodenum
  – Usually relatively large (> 1 cm)
– Mucosa: may show erosion, ulceration

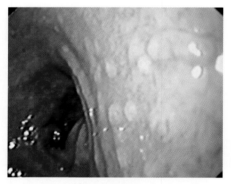

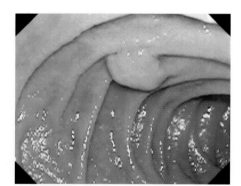

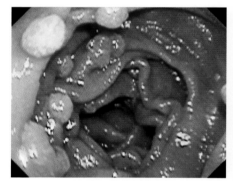

Fig. 3.**149** **Villous adenomas and polypoid lesions in bulbitis**
a Small villous adenoma

b Villous adenoma

c Multiple villous adenomas

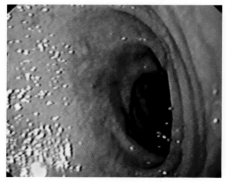

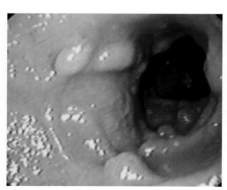

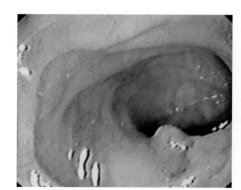

d Bulbitis

e, f Erosions in the duodenal bulb

f

Sprue, Crohn Disease, and Whipple Disease

■ Sprue

Sprue is an immune-mediated condition in which the mucosa of the small bowel becomes damaged due to the ingestion of gluten-containing foods. The disease is characterized by the loss of mucosal villi, resulting in malabsorption and diarrhea. Involvement of the duodenum is almost always present.

■ Diagnosis

 Endoscopic diagnostic criteria (Figs. 3.**150**, 3.**151**)

▶ Mucosa appears grossly unchanged in some cases
▶ Erythema
▶ Abnormally smooth mucosa
▶ Loss of mucosal granularity
▶ Effacement of valvulae conniventes
▶ Mucosal atrophy

Differential diagnosis

▶ Tropical sprue
▶ Eosinophilic gastroenteritis
▶ Lymphoma
▶ Viral gastroenteritis

Checklist for endoscopic evaluation

▶ Deep duodenoscopy
▶ Evaluate mucosa and valvulae conniventes

Additional Studies

▶ Biopsy distal to the papilla
▶ Gliadin antibodies
▶ Small bowel function studies (D-xylose test, lactose H2 breath test)

Comments

The macroscopic and histological findings are very typical. The diagnosis is considered established if the complaints subside after gluten is eliminated from the diet. The risk of developing an intestinal lymphoma or carcinoma is high in untreated cases of sprue.

■ Crohn Disease

The lesions of Crohn disease can also involve the duodenum, but this occurs in fewer than 5% of patients (Fig. 3.**152**).

 Endoscopy reveals small, aphthoid erosions and ulcerations.

■ Whipple Disease

Whipple disease is a very rare, bacterial systemic disease that is characterized by joint pain, weight loss, and diarrhea. Swollen

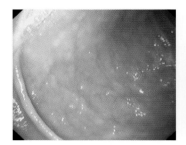

Fig. 3.**150** **Villous atrophy in sprue**

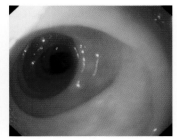

Fig. 3.**151 a–c** **Duodenum in sprue**

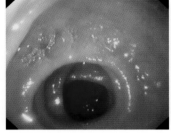

b

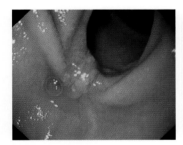

a

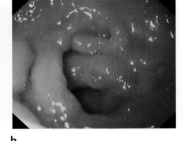

b

Fig. 3.**152 a–c** **Crohn disease of the duodenum**

c

villi, thickened bowel wall, and edema are found in affected segments of the duodenum and jejunum. The histological findings are diagnostic.

 At endoscopy, the mucosa is fragile with a whitish speckled pattern. The villi appear blunted and swollen.

Duodenal Diverticula

Although duodenal diverticula are not uncommon and are discovered in up to 20 % of autopsies, they are rarely seen at endoscopy. They are detected more frequently by radiography (Fig. 3.**155**). The frequency of endoscopic detection increases when a side-viewing duodenoscope is used.

■ Clinical Aspects

Duodenal diverticula usually cause no complaints, although some cases present with biliary tract obstruction or symptoms due to impacted food residues.

■ Location

Duodenal diverticula are found predominantly in the medial wall of the descending duodenum, usually at the Vater papilla or at the opening of an accessory pancreatic duct (Fig. 3.**153**).

■ Diagnosis

 Endoscopic diagnostic criteria (Fig. 3.**154**)
▶ Outpouching of the duodenal wall
▶ Pouch may contain food residues

Differential diagnosis
▶ Typical appearance

Checklist for endoscopic evaluation
▶ Location
▶ Size

Additional Studies
▶ Upper GI contrast series for accurate size determination (Fig. 3.**155**)

Comments
Treatment is usually unnecessary. With obstruction of the biliary tract or duodenum, operative treatment is required.

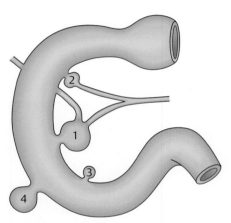

Fig. 3.**153** **Sites of occurrence of duodenal diverticula**
1 Juxtapapillary
2 At an accessory papilla
3 Medial wall of the inferior flexure
4 Lateral wall of the inferior flexure

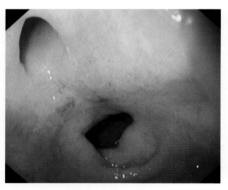 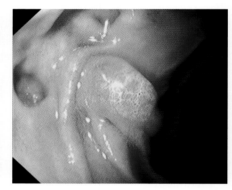

Fig. 3.**154** **Duodenal diverticulum**
a Bulbar diverticulum
b Diverticulum next to the papilla

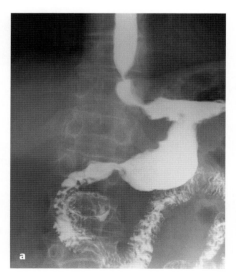

Fig. 3.**155** **Duodenal diverticula in upper GI contrast radiographs**
a Juxtapapillary diverticulum
b Diverticulum in the medial wall of the inferior flexure

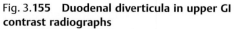

Duodenal Changes Associated with Diseases in Adjacent Organs

■ Adjacent Organs

The duodenum is related in its course to the liver, gallbladder, pancreas, right colic flexure, and kidney (Fig. 3.**156**). Diseases of these organs can lead to endoscopically detectable changes in the duodenum.

 Endoscopic features

▶ **Liver**
  - Metastases: indentation of the bulb
  - Cysts: indentation of the bulb
▶ **Gallbladder**
  - Hydrops: indentation of the duodenum
  - Cholecystitis: edema of the duodenal wall
▶ **Bile ducts**
  - Klatskin tumor: duodenal stenosis
▶ **Pancreas** (Figs. 3.**157**, 3.**158**)
  - Chronic pancreatitis: lymphedema
  - Acute pancreatitis: compression
  - Tumor: infiltration

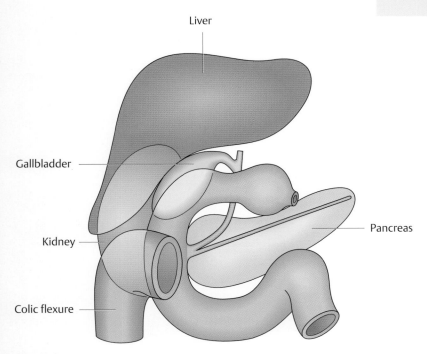

Fig. 3.**156** **Relations of the duodenum**

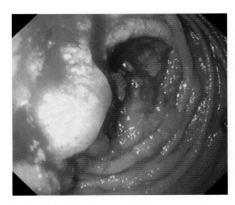

Fig. 3.**157** **Carcinoma of the pancreatic head infiltrating the duodenum**

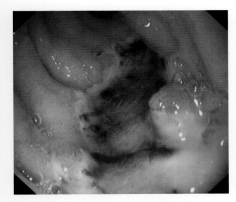

Fig. 3.**158** **Duodenum in necrotizing pancreatitis**
a Acute pancreatitis with inflammatory change and necrosis in the duodenum

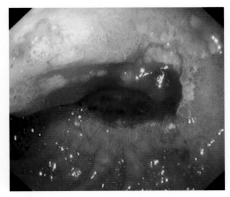

b Necrotizing pancreatitis with marked inflammatory changes and hemorrhages in the duodenum

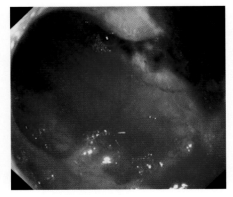

c Necrotizing pancreatitis with infiltration of the duodenum

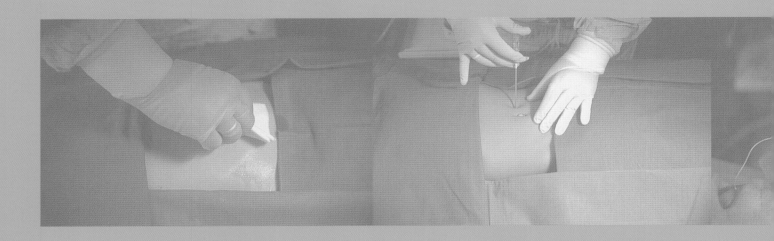

4 Interventional Procedures and Extended Endoscopic Examination Methods

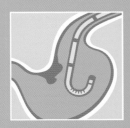

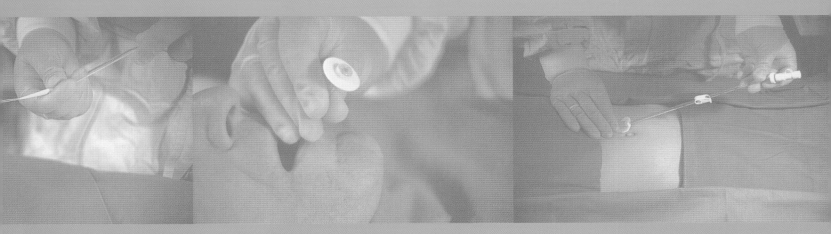

Overview of Interventional Endoscopy

Table 4.1 Interventional procedures in esophagogastroduodenoscopy (EGD)

- ▶ Endoscopic hemostasis
- ▶ Specimen collection
- ▶ Endoscopic treatment of precancerous lesions and early carcinoma
- ▶ Endoscopic tube placement
- ▶ Foreign body removal
- ▶ Endoscopic treatment of stenoses
- ▶ Dye methods

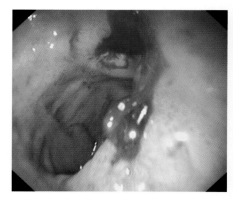

Fig. 4.**1**   Bleeding gastric ulcer

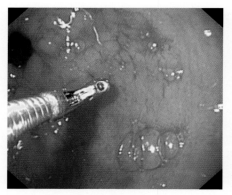

Fig. 4.**2**   Endoscopic biopsy

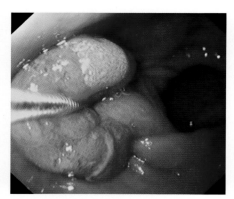

Fig. 4.**3**   Polyp removal

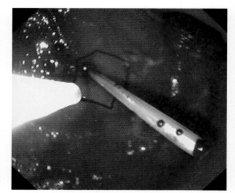

Fig. 4.**4**   PEG placement

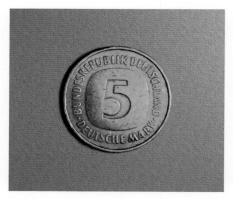

Fig. 4.**5**   Foreign body removal: coins

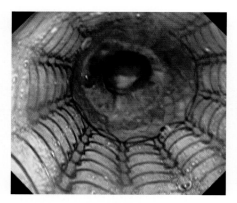

Fig. 4.**6**   Stent insertion for a malignant esophageal stricture

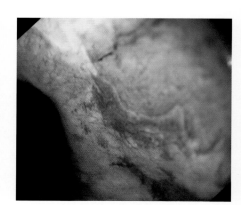

Fig. 4.**7**   Methylene blue staining of Barrett esophagus

Upper Gastrointestinal Bleeding: Incidence and Signs

■ Incidence

Acute gastrointestinal bleeding is the most common emergency in gastroenterology. Ninety percent of all acute hemorrhages arise in the upper gastrointestinal tract, approximately 9% in the colon, and approximately 1% between the ligament of Treitz and the ileocecal valve (Figs. 4.8, 4.9). The incidence is age-dependent, ranging from approximately 30 : 100 000 in young individuals to as much as 400 : 100 000 in persons over age 75 according to published reports. The overall mortality rate is approximately 15%; it is markedly lower in young patients, rising to 40% in elderly patients with multiple morbidity.

■ Causes

The most frequent cause is ulcer bleeding associated with the ingestion of nonsteroidal anti-inflammatory drugs (NSAIDs). This type of bleeding usually occurs early during NSAID use and may occur even at low doses. The concomitant use of corticosteroids significantly increases the risk, and concurrent anticoagulant use can increase it dramatically.

■ Symptoms

The main symptoms of upper gastrointestinal bleeding are hematemesis, melena, and signs of hemorrhagic shock.

The major problems associated with upper gastrointestinal bleeding are hemorrhagic shock and aspiration pneumonia (bleeding and vomiting). They dictate the priorities that are followed in primary treatment:

1. Hemodynamic stabilization
2. Maintenance of adequate respiration
3. Identifying the source of bleeding and hemostasis
4. Prevention of rebleeding

Table 4.**2**   **Upper gastrointestinal bleeding**

Cardinal symptoms and likelihood of massive bleeding	
Hematemesis	20%
Melena	5–10%
Hematochezia (red blood in the stool)	

General symptoms
▶ Dizziness
▶ Syncope
▶ Dyspnea
▶ Angina pectoris
▶ Hemorrhagic shock

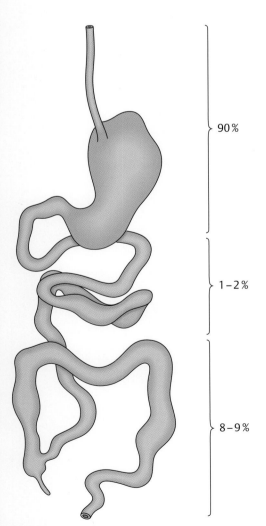

Fig. 4.**8**   **Relative frequency of acute bleeding at different levels in the gastrointestinal tract**

90%

1–2%

8–9%

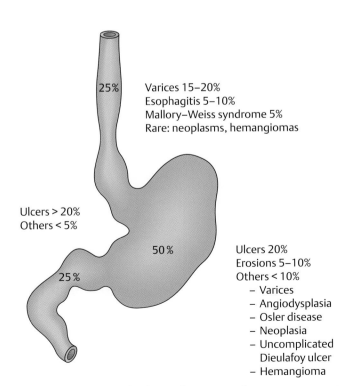

25%

Varices 15–20%
Esophagitis 5–10%
Mallory–Weiss syndrome 5%
Rare: neoplasms, hemangiomas

Ulcers > 20%
Others < 5%

50%

25%

Ulcers 20%
Erosions 5–10%
Others < 10%
  – Varices
  – Angiodysplasia
  – Osler disease
  – Neoplasia
  – Uncomplicated
    Dieulafoy ulcer
  – Hemangioma

Fig. 4.**9**   **Location and relative frequency of acute upper gastrointestinal bleeding**

Upper Gastrointestinal Bleeding: Primary Treatment

■ Hemodynamic Stabilization

► Is there impending or frank hemorrhagic shock (Table 4.**3**)?
► **Caution:** Symptoms may be masked by:
– Beta-blocking drugs
– Vasovagal bradycardia
– Preexisting hypertension
► **Note:**
– An orthostatic rise in the heart rate by more than 20 bpm suggests a blood loss greater than 500 mL.
– A blood pressure differential > 15–20 mmHg between sitting and lying down suggests a blood loss greater than 1000 mL.
► **Treat for shock before performing endoscopy!**
– Place two large-caliber i. v. lines as soon as possible.
– Augment the circulating volume (preferably with a crystalloid such as 100 mL physiological saline solution or Ringer lactate).
– Goal: Heart rate < 100 bpm, blood pressure > 100 mmHg
► Necessary laboratory tests
– Blood for typing, cross-matched blood, blood count, coagulation values, electrolytes

Table 4.3 Impending hemorrhagic shock

► Heart rate > 100
► Blood pressure < 100 systolic
► Cool extremities
► Cold sweat
► Obtundation
► Angina pectoris

■ Maintaining Adequate Respiration

► Clear the airway (**Caution:** vomited blood).
► Suction the airway as needed.
► Administer O_2 by nasal catheter.
► Intubate if necessary (Table 4.**4**).

Table 4.4 Indications for intubation

► Frank hemorrhagic shock
► Patient somnolent before endoscopy
► Patient uncooperative before endoscopy

■ Identify the Source of Bleeding and Stop the Bleeding

► Preendoscopy checklist
– Adequate treatment for shock?
– Need to intubate before endoscopy?
– Time for blood replacement? (If Hb < 8, try to transfuse before endoscopy.)
– Open surgery instead of endoscopy (Table 4.**5**)?

► Identify the source of bleeding
– Always perform complete esophagogastroduodenoscopy (EGD) according to standard protocols.
– If one bleeding site is detected, always look for another potential source of bleeding.
– It is not unusual for multiple sources of bleeding to coexist.
► Hemostasis
– The most frequent sources of upper gastrointestinal bleeding are ulcers and varices (Fig. 4.**9**).
– Hemostatic modalities include pharmacological therapy, balloon catheter insertion, injection therapy, thermal methods, banding, and transjugular intrahepatic portosystemic shunting (TIPS). The method of choice is determined by customary recommendations and by the technical capabilities and interests of the endoscopy department.
– The goals of endoscopic treatment are always to control active bleeding and prevent rebleeding. Endoscopic techniques are appropriate for the sources of bleeding listed in Table 4.**6**. Necessary instruments and equipment are listed in Table 4.**7**.
► Prevent rebleeding

Table 4.5 Indications for open surgery instead of endoscopy

► Refractory shock
► Recurrent bleeding from a known ulcer on the posterior wall of the duodenal bulb
► Recurrent bleeding in an elderly patient with comorbidity
► Recurrent bleeding in a patient with high initial bleeding activity

Table 4.6 Indications for endoscopic hemostasis

► Esophageal varices and fundic varices
► Gastric and duodenal ulcer
► Reflux esophagitis
► Mallory–Weiss syndrome
► Erosions

Table 4.7 Necessary emergency instruments and equipment

► Endoscope with a large working channel
► High-performance suction pump
► Second suction pump for the pharynx
► Water pump for irrigation
► Sclerotherapy needles
► Injection needles for Histoacryl
► Clips with applicators
► Argon plasma coagulation
► Multiband ligator set
► Epinephrine 1 : 1000
► Histoacryl
► Lipiodol
► Polydocanol 1 %
► Fibrin glue (optional)

Bleeding Esophageal Varices and Fundic Varices: Medications and Tubes

The mortality rate due to variceal bleeding (Fig. 4.**10**) is high, at 15–30%. The recurrence rate after an initial bleed is approximately 60% during the first two weeks. One third of varices will stop bleeding spontaneously.

■ Treatment Methods

The following treatment methods are used:

- Pharmacological
  - Terlipressin plus nitrate
- Balloon tamponade
  - Sengstaken–Blakemore tube (for esophageal varices)
  - Linton–Nachlas tube (for fundic varices)
- Endoscopic
  - Sclerotherapy
  - Banding
- TIPS
- Operative treatment

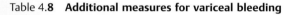

Fig. 4.**10** **Bleeding esophageal varices**

Besides the control of bleeding and prevention of rebleeding, additional therapeutic measures may be taken depending on the clinical situation (Table 4.**8**).

Table 4.**8** **Additional measures for variceal bleeding**

> - PPI i. v.
> - Antibiotic therapy (lowers risk of rebleeding and of spontaneous bacterial peritonitis)
> - Lactulose 3 x 50 mL
> - Neomycin 2–4 g/day
> - Protein restriction
> - Fresh frozen plasma
> - Packed red blood cells
> - Volume replacement

■ Pharmacological Therapy of Bleeding Esophageal Varices

Principle and Key Characteristics

- Principle: medication to lower the portal venous and intravenous pressure
- Vasopressin and terlipressin are the only two medications that have been approved for the treatment of bleeding esophageal varices.
  - Terlipressin is superior to vasopressin owing to its longer half-life.
  - Terlipressin should be combined with nitrates due to possible side effects (ischemia and necrosis).
- Pharmacologic therapy is an acceptable alternative to balloon tamponade if emergency endoscopy cannot be performed.

Materials

- Terlipressin
- Glyceryl nitrate
- Intravenous access
- Perfusor and perfusor tubing
- Syringes

Technique

- Terlipressin, 2 mg by i. v. bolus
- Repeat at 1 mg every four to six hours
- Duration: two to three days
- Always combined with glyceryl nitrate i. v. by perfusor, 1–4 mg/hour

■ Balloon Tamponade

Principle and Key Characteristics

- Principle: external compression of the bleeding varix with an inflated balloon
- Suitable if emergency endoscopy is not an option or as a temporizing measure after unsuccessful endoscopic or operative treatment or TIPS
- Esophageal varices: Sengstaken–Blakemore tube (two balloons)
- Fundic varices: Linton–Nachlas tube (one balloon)

Problems

- Pressure necrosis
- Aspiration pneumonia
- Rupture of the cardia
- Retching or vomiting may dislodge the tube, causing airway obstruction (Tube can be cut in an emergency; keep scissors handy)

Materials

- Sengstaken–Blakemore or Linton–Nachlas tube
- Topical anesthetic
- Lubricant
- Padding
- Adhesive tape
- Manometer
- 50-mL syringe
- Clamps

Technique

- Do not tamponade if the patient is vomiting.
- Check the tube for air tightness before use.
- Smear the tube and balloon with lubricant.
- Anesthetize the nasal mucosa.
- Squeeze residual air from the balloon.
- Insert the tube transnasally, advancing to 50 cm.
- **Sengstaken–Blakemore tube**
  - Inflate the gastric balloon to 150 mL and clamp off. Slowly withdraw the tube until a springy resistance, synchronous with respirations, is felt.
  - Secure the tube with strong adhesive tape.
  - Pad the tube at the nostrils.
  - Inflate the epithelial balloon to 45 mmHg by manometry, then clamp.
- **Linton–Nachlas tube**
  - Inflate the balloon to 400 mL.
  - Withdraw until a springy resistance is felt.
  - Secure in place.
  - Add another 200 mL.
- Deflate the tube for 30 minutes every six to eight hours.
- Maximum duration of tube placement: 24 hours.

Bleeding Esophageal Varices: Sclerotherapy

Endoscopic Treatments

The treatment of choice for bleeding varices is endoscopic therapy. The following methods are available:
- Sclerotherapy with polidocanol (esophageal varices)
- Rubber band ligation (esophageal varices)
- Sclerotherapy with Histoacryl (fundic varices)

Sclerotherapy with Polidocanol (Ethoxysclerol)

Principle and Key Characteristics (Fig. 4.11)
- Principle: compression and thrombosis of the varix, induction of inflammation with subsequent scarring
- Paravariceal or intravariceal injection
- Established therapy
- Advantages
  - Good in cases where vision is poor
  - Relatively easy to perform

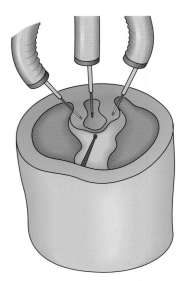

Fig. 4.**11** **Treatment of esophageal varices**. Principle of paravariceal and intravariceal injection of the sclerosant

Materials
- Endoscope
- Suction pump
- Water jet
- Sclerotherapy needle, 4–6 mm long
- Polidocanol 0.5–1 %

 Technique (Figs. 4.**12**, 4.**13**)
- Lateral position with the upper body elevated
- No pharyngeal anesthesia
- Pulse oximetry
- The instrument is inserted, and the bleeding varix is identified.
- Injection is begun close to the cardia.
- Intravariceal and paravariceal injection
  - 0.5 mL injected on both sides of the varix (produces compression, inflammation, fibrosis)
  - 1.0 mL injected directly into the varix (induces thrombosis)
  - Maximum of 2 mL per injection site
- If there is postinjection bleeding, advance the endoscope and compress the varix for approximately one minute.
- If no further bleeding occurs, sclerose any varices that show signs of an increased bleeding risk.
- If treatment is unsuccessful, discontinue sclerotherapy and insert a Sengstaken–Blakemore tube.

Aftercare
- See Management of Bleeding Varices, page 88.

Complications
- Sclerotherapy ulcer
- Esophageal stricture
- Esophageal perforation
- Pleural effusion

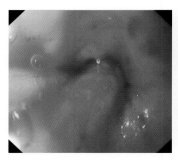 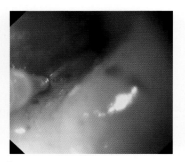 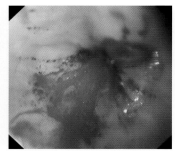 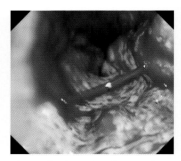

Fig. 4.**12 a–c** **Injection therapy of bleeding esophageal varices**   b   c

Fig. 4.**13** **Spurting hemorrhage from an esophageal varix**

Bleeding Esophageal Varices: Banding

Principle and Key Characteristics

- ▶ Varix is sucked into a sleeve at the endoscope tip and ligated with an elastic band.
- ▶ Induction of thrombosis, necrosis, and scarring
- ▶ Established therapy
- ▶ Advantages
  - Low complication rate
  - Overall mortality and mortality due to bleeding are lower than in sclerotherapy
  - Early rebleeding is less common than with sclerotherapy
- ▶ Disadvantage
  - Limited vision in cases with massive bleeding

Materials (Fig. 4.14 a)

- ▶ Endoscope
- ▶ Suction pump
- ▶ Water jet
- ▶ Variceal ligation set (multi- or single-band ligator)

 Technique (Figs. 4.14 b, 4.15)

- ▶ Use a standard endoscope with an overtube.
- ▶ Advance the overtube.
- ▶ Perform a complete EGD.
- ▶ Withdraw the endoscope.
- ▶ Set up the endoscopic and ligation set.
- ▶ Reenter through the overtube.
- ▶ Begin the ligation near the cardia.

- ▶ Entrap the varix, suck the varix into the sleeve, and release the elastic band.
- ▶ Usually three or four bands are applied per sitting, but considerably more may be placed if needed.
- ▶ If bleeding is severe and it is difficult to identify the source, band the distal varices.

Aftercare

- ▶ Repeat three or four times at two-week intervals.
- ▶ Reexamine at three months.

Complications

- ▶ Early: perforation of the hypopharynx or esophagus by the overtube
- ▶ Late: strictures, stenoses

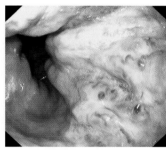

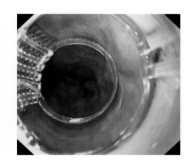

Fig. 4.**15** **Banding of esophageal varices**
a   The varix is identified

b   The endoscope is advanced

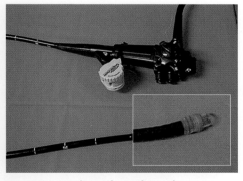

Fig. 4.**14** **Banding of esophageal varices**
a   Endoscope prepared for banding, with a close-up view of the endoscope tip

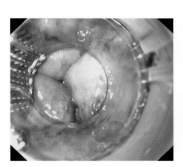

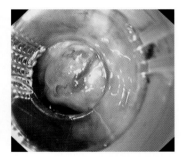

c   The tip of the sleeve is placed over the varix

d   The varix is sucked into the sleeve

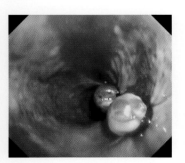

b   Banded esophageal varix

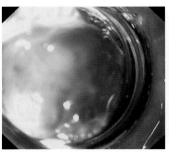

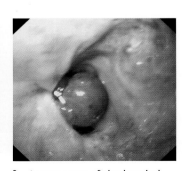

e   The elastic band is released

f   Appearance of the banded varix

Sclerotherapy of Fundic Varices, TIPS, and Operative Treatment

Interventional Procedures

Principle and Key Characteristics

▶ Principle: The varices are obliterated with a tissue adhesive.
▶ Sclerotherapy with cyanoacrylate (Histoacryl) is the treatment of choice for fundic varices (Fig. 4.**16**).

Materials

▶ Endoscope
▶ Suction pumps
▶ Water jet
▶ Disposable sclerotherapy needles, 6 mm long with 0.7 mm outer diameter
▶ Histoacryl
▶ Lipiodol
▶ Protective eyewear
▶ Distilled water
▶ Silicone oil

 Technique

▶ Use protective eyewear.
▶ Draw Histoacryl and Lipiodol (1:1) into a 2-mL syringe.
▶ Flush the sclerotherapy needle with distilled water (Histoacryl polymerizes on contact with electrolytes).
▶ Introduce silicone oil into the working channel.
▶ Insert the syringe.
▶ Inject 0.5–1 mL into the varix.
▶ Flush with water.
▶ Retract the needle into the plastic sleeve, and wait one minute for the Histoacryl to polymerize before completely withdrawing the needle through the endoscope.
▶ If this is unsuccessful, insert a Linton–Nachlas tube.

Complications

▶ Histoacryl embolism
▶ Sclerotherapy ulcer

■ Transjugular Intrahepatic Portosystemic Shunt (TIPS)

Principle and Key Characteristics (Fig. 4.**17**)

▶ Principle: A connection is established between the hepatic vein and intrahepatic portal vein branch.
▶ A puncture needle is passed to the right hepatic vein through a transjugular catheter, and the intrahepatic portal vein branch is punctured. The puncture tract is dilated and then stabilized with an expanding stent.
▶ Last recourse for refractory bleeding.

■ Operative Treatment

Principle and Key Characteristics

▶ Principle: surgical creation of a portosystemic anastomosis.
▶ Not practical in emergency situations.
▶ Considerably higher mortality compared with TIPS.

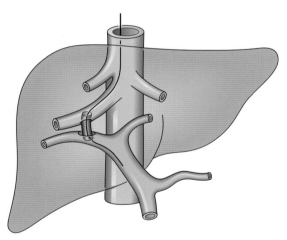

Fig. 4.**17** **Schematic diagram of TIPS placement.** The shunt establishes a connection between the hepatic vein and portal vein

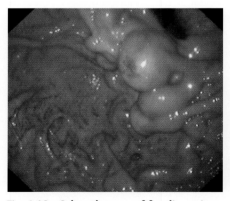
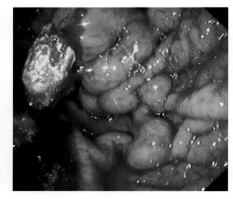
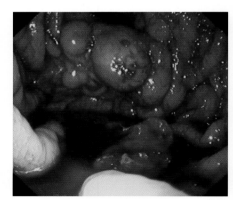

Fig. 4.**16** **Sclerotherapy of fundic varices with Histoacryl**
a The presumed bleeding site is identified (varix with a "red spot")

b Histoacryl is injected

c Appearance after sclerotherapy

Bleeding Ulcers: Nonoperative Therapies

■ Incidence and Symptoms

Fifty percent of all acute upper gastrointestinal hemorrhages are caused by a bleeding ulcer (Fig. 4.**18**). It is estimated that approximately 20% of all patients with recurrent gastric or duodenal ulcers experience bleeding. This may be an oozing hemorrhage with gradual progression of anemia or may present as an acute, massive, life-threatening hemorrhage.

The symptoms are variable and may be very subtle, particularly in NSAID users. Approximately 80% of bleeding ulcers will stop bleeding spontaneously, and 20% of those will rebleed. The mortality rate is 6–15%. Acute bleeding can be successfully controlled by endoscopic treatment in over 85% of cases. The risk of recurrence after primary hemostasis is 20–25%.

■ Nonoperative Treatment Methods

The following nonoperative treatment modalities are used:
► Pharmacological therapy
► Endoscopic techniques
  – Injection therapy: epinephrine, physiological saline solution, polidocanol, ethanol, fibrin glue
  – Hemostatic clips
  – Thermal methods: laser, electrocoagulation, argon plasma coagulation

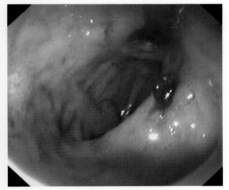

Fig. 4.**18** **Bleeding gastric ulcer**

■ Indications for Endoscopic Treatment

The Forrest classification is used in selecting patients for endoscopic treatment (Table 4.**9**; Figs. 4.**19**, 4.**20**). Treatment is indicated for Forrest classes Ia and Ib, which are actively bleeding lesions, and for a high percentage of recurrent ulcers of class IIa. For class IIb lesions, an effort is made to flush away the adherent clot. If this is successful, the treatment decision is based on the new finding. Removing the clot may induce active bleeding, leave a "visible vessel," or expose a hematin- or fibrin-covered ulcer base.

If the bleeding cannot be controlled endoscopically, prompt operative treatment is indicated.

Table 4.**9** **Forrest classification**

Class	Bleeding activity	Risk of rebleeding (%)
I	**Active bleeding**	
Ia	Spurting hemorrhage	90
Ib	Oozing hemorrhage	30
II	**Signs of hemorrhage without active bleeding**	
IIa	Visible vessel	50–100
IIb	Adherent clot	20
IIc	Hematin on ulcer base	< 5
III	**Ulcer base with no signs of bleeding**	< 5

Forrest Class I–IIa lesions are an indication for endoscopic treatment

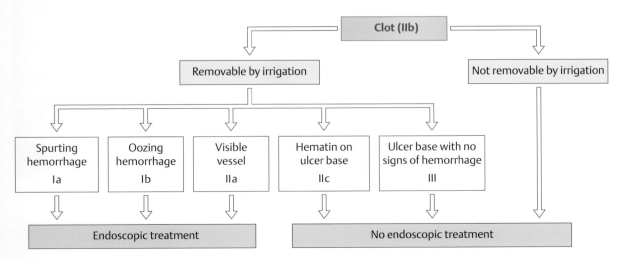

Fig. 4.**19** **Flowchart for management of an adherent clot**

Bleeding Ulcers: Forrest Classification

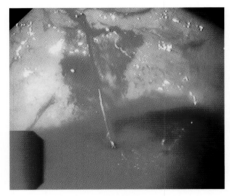

Fig. 4.20   Forrest classification of acute ulcer bleeding
a Class Ia: spurting hemorrhage

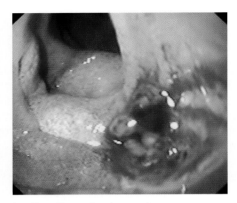

b Class Ib: oozing hemorrhage

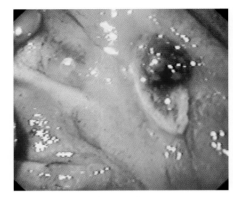

c Class IIa: visible vessel

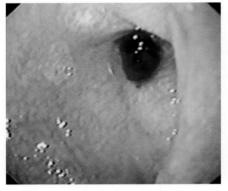

d Class IIb: clot adherent to the ulcer

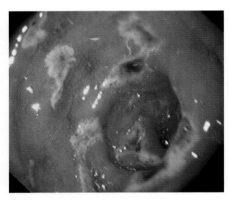

e Class IIc: hematin on the ulcer

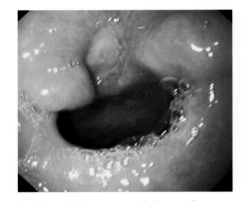

f Class III: fibrin-covered ulcer with no signs of hemorrhage

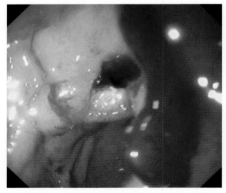

Fig. 4.21   Epinephrine injection for acute ulcer bleeding
a Two bleeding ulcers (smaller one at the center, larger one at approximately the 5-o'clock position)

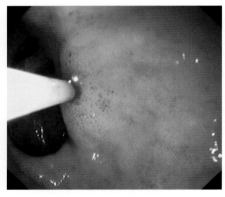

b Epinephrine is injected around the base of the larger ulcer

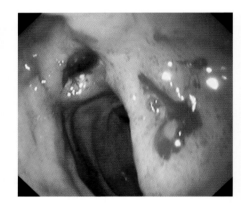

c Appearance after injection

Bleeding Ulcers: Pharmacological Therapy and Injection Techniques

■ Pharmacological Therapy of Bleeding Ulcers

Hemostasis cannot be achieved with medical therapy alone. PPI are used, but their benefit is still unproved. If *H. pylori* is detected, eradication therapy should be performed. This can expedite healing and lower the risk of recurrence. NSAIDs should be discontinued.

■ Endoscopic Techniques

The treatment of choice is endoscopic hemostasis (injection therapy, hemoclips, thermal methods).

■ Injection Therapy

Key Characteristics

▶ Epinephrine
  - Therapy of choice
  - Safe, economical, can be used to treat rebleeding after prior hemostasis with polidocanol
▶ Polidocanol
  - Very effective, especially after initial use of epinephrine
  - Problem: enlarges tissue lesion, should not be used to treat rebleeding
  - Agent of second choice
▶ Fibrin glue
  - Two components (fibrin and thrombin) form a fibrin clot when mixed together. They are mixed at the time of injection.
  - Excellent tissue compatibility; very costly, laborious technique
  - Very effective for rebleeding
▶ Physiological saline solution, glucose, ethanol
  - Very rarely used today as a solitary treatment

Materials

▶ Endoscope
▶ Suction pumps
▶ Water jet
▶ Single-lumen injection needles for epinephrine and polidocanol, double-lumen needles for fibrin glue
▶ Epinephrine 1 : 10 000 in physiological saline solution, 1 % polidocanol, fibrin glue

Technique

▶ Epinephrine (Fig. 4.**21**)
  - Make several injections of 1 mL each around the bleeding ulcer.
  - Then inject 1–2 mL into the bleeding site at the ulcer base.
▶ Polidocanol
  - Inject 1 mL of polidocanol into the bleeding site.
  - **Caution:** Inject no more than 2 mL per ulcer; more could cause a substantial tissue lesion.
▶ Fibrin glue
  - Preflush the needle with physiological saline solution.
  - Inject 2 mL of both components into the bleeding site through a double-lumen needle.
  - Then flush the needle with physiological saline solution.

4

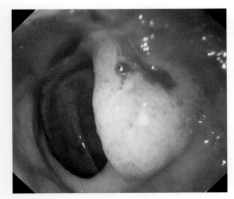

d Appearance after irrigation

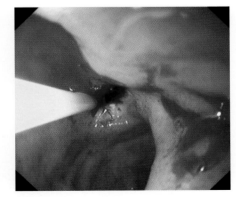

e Epinephrine is injected around the base of the smaller ulcer

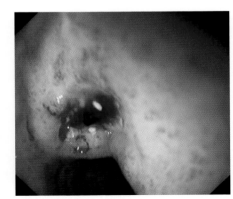

f Appearance after injection

Bleeding Ulcers: Hemoclip Application and Thermal Methods

Interventional Procedures

■ Hemoclip Application

Principle and Key Characteristics

▶ Principle: compression of the lesion or bleeding vessel with a metal clip
▶ Safe, appears as effective as injection therapy, causes no tissue damage, relatively low cost
▶ Excellent for treating "visible vessels" and arterial hemorrhages, Dieulafoy ulcer, and bleeding after polypectomies

Materials

▶ Endoscope
▶ Suction pumps
▶ Water jet
▶ Hemoclips with applicator

 Technique
▶ Load the hemoclip onto the applicator and insert.
▶ Apply the hemoclip to the bleeding vessel.

■ Thermal Methods

Key Characteristics

▶ Several options: electrocoagulation, laser, argon plasma coagulation
▶ No more effective than injection methods, rarely used alone
▶ Argon plasma coagulation: shallow penetration, very effective for oozing (Fig. 4.**24**)

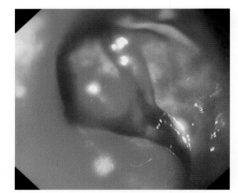

Fig. 4.22 Clipping of a bleeding gastric ulcer
a The bleeding site is identified

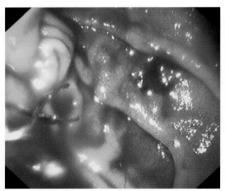

b The applicator is advanced to the bleeding site. The open clip is visible on the left side of the image

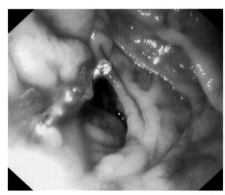

c The clip is applied, largely controlling the hemorrhage

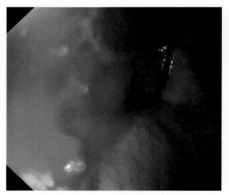

Fig. 4.23 Clipping of a bleeding biopsy site
a Brisk bleeding after a tissue biopsy

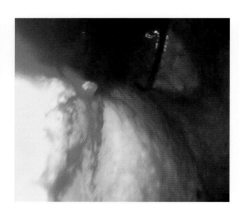

b Appearance after irrigation

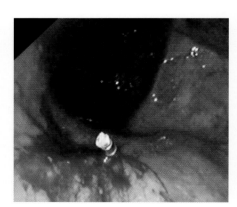

c After hemoclip application

Bleeding Ulcers: Management after Primary Hemostasis and in Special Cases

■ Management after Primary Hemostasis

Figure 4.25 outlines the follow-through regimen after primary hemostasis has been achieved. Scheduling an early repeat endoscopy does not improve the prognosis. When rebleeding occurs after primary hemostasis, the success rate of repeat endoscopic hemostasis is 50–70%.

■ Hemostasis of a Mallory–Weiss Lesion

A Mallory–Weiss lesion (Fig. 4.26 a) is infiltrated with epinephrine diluted 1:10 000 in physiological saline solution, or it may be obliterated with fibrin glue.

■ Hemostasis of a Bleeding Dieulafoy Ulcer

The methods of choice are epinephrine injection and hemoclip application.

■ Hemostasis in Hemorrhagic Gastritis

Hemorrhagic gastritis (Fig. 4.26 b) usually does not require specific endoscopic hemostasis. It can be adequately managed with PPI.

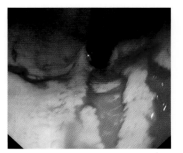

Fig. 4.26
a Bleeding Mallory–Weiss lesion

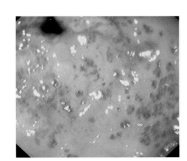

b Hemorrhagic gastritis

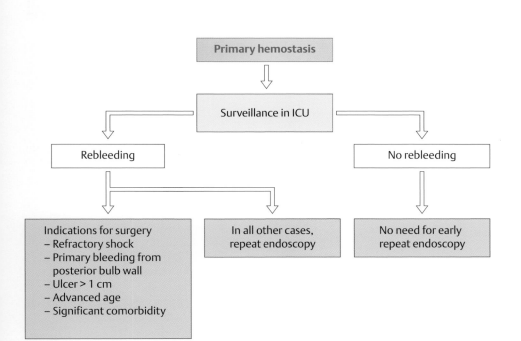

Fig. 4.25 Follow-through after primary hemostasis

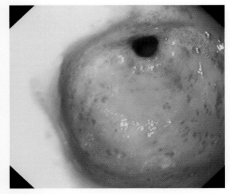 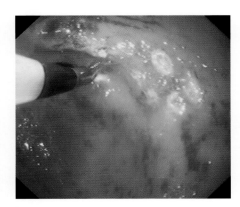 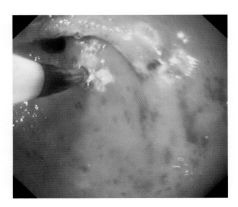

Fig. 4.24 a–c Argon plasma coagulation in GAVE syndrome

b

c

Specimen Collection

Indications

Endoscopy is the ideal medium for the selective collection of tissue and fluid specimens for further analysis. The risk of bleeding or perforation is minimal when some very simple rules are followed.

Whenever gastroscopy is performed, biopsy specimens should be taken from the gastric antrum for *H. pylori* detection. The degree of sampling from normal-appearing mucosa will vary greatly from one examiner to the next.

Additionally, of course, all abnormal-appearing mucosal areas that cannot be classified by gross inspection should be biopsied, with due regard for contraindications. The endoscopic specimens are sent for histological, microbiological, or other testing (polymerase chain reaction [PCR], etc.).

Procedures

The methods most commonly used to collect specimens during EGD are as follows:

▶ Biopsy
▶ Brush cytology
▶ Fluid sampling

■ Biopsy

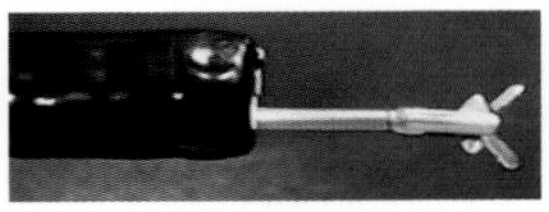

Indications

▶ Any normal-appearing antral mucosa (and gastric body mucosa) for *H. pylori* detection
▶ Any abnormal-appearing area that cannot be positively classified by gross inspection

Fig. 4.**27**   **Biopsy forceps**

Contraindications

▶ Coagulation defect (coumarin use, hepatic cirrhosis); the use of aspirin and other NSAIDs is not a contraindication.
▶ Planned enucleation of a submucosal tumor
▶ In the area of diverticula
▶ In the area of varices
▶ In areas of radiation-induced esophagitis

Techniques

▶ **Simple forceps biopsy**
  – Forceps jaws come in various designs (large, small, sharp, blunt, with or without a central prong, etc.) for use in different situations (Fig. 4.**27**).
▶ **Buttonhole biopsy**
  – Used to sample tissue from submucosal masses.
  – First the mucosa over the mass is resected, then a deeper specimen is taken from the submucosal lesion.
  – Indication: submucosal mass
  – Complications: bleeding, perforation
  – **Caution:** This type of biopsy is contraindicated if tumor enucleation is planned.

▶ **Suction biopsy**
  – The biopsy tube is passed endoscopically into the second part of the duodenum; tissue is sucked into the port, cut off with a sliding blade, and retained in a trap.
  – Formerly used to sample tissue in cases of suspected celiac disease. Today has been largely superseded by forceps biopsy due to the substantial perforation risk.

■ Brush Cytology

Indications

▶ Larger lesions that are difficult to sample adequately with biopsy forceps (e.g., strictures)
▶ Adjunct to biopsy in Barrett epithelium

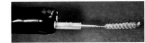

Fig. 4.**28**   **Brush attachment for endoscopic brush cytology**

Contraindications

▶ Coagulation defect
▶ **Caution:** The bristles of an endoscopic brush have significant traumatic potential and can cause considerable bleeding!

Technique

▶ The brush (Fig. 4.**28**) is rubbed repeatedly across the suspicious lesion, retracted into the guide sleeve, and both are withdrawn through the endoscope channel.
▶ The material is wiped onto glass slides and air-dried.

■ Fluid Sampling

Indications

▶ pH determination of the gastric juice (e.g., to assess response to PPI therapy)
▶ Obtaining material for microbiological testing (e.g., *Giardia* in duodenal secretions)

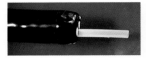

Fig. 4.**29**   **Tube for fluid sampling**

Contraindications

▶ None

Technique

▶ The sampling tube (Fig. 4.**29**) is passed down the working channel of the endoscope, and a fluid sample is aspirated with a syringe.
▶ The specimen is processed according to requirements.

Endoscopic Treatment of Precancerous Lesions and Early Carcinoma

Both open resection and endoscopic techniques are available for the treatment of precancerous lesions and early carcinomas of the esophagus and stomach.

■ Open Resection

The advantages of open resection are that it permits a more radical tumor removal and allows for extensive histological processing and evaluation of the excised tissue.

Disadvantages include problems associated with the postoperative defect, the operative mortality and morbidity, and the limitations that are frequently imposed by coexisting illnesses.

■ Endoscopic Treatments

Endoscopic treatment options include polypectomy, endoscopic mucosectomy, and photodynamic therapy. Endoscopic polypectomy is a long-established procedure, while mucosectomy and photodynamic therapy have been increasingly performed in recent years.

■ Polypectomy

Key Characteristics

▶ The polyp is snared with a wire loop and transected at the base with high-frequency diathermy.

Indication

▶ Gastric and duodenal polyps that are 10 mm or larger in diameter

Contraindications

▶ Coagulation defect (Quick prothrombin time [PT]: < 50 %, platelets: < 50 000/µL)
▶ Aspirin use
▶ Intramural tumors

 Technique

▶ Preprocedure checklist
  – Informed consent?
  – Coagulation studies?
  – Aspirin discontinued five days before procedure?
  – Emergency instruments and equipment available?
▶ Preparations
  – Place the neutral electrode on the patient's thigh.
  – Set up the high-frequency diathermy unit.
  – Check the function of the polypectomy snare.
▶ Polyp removal
  – Visualize the polyp.
  – For a larger polyp, infiltrate the base with epinephrine or secure it with a clip.
  – Place the open snare over the polyp, and tighten the snare under vision.
  – Gently lift the snared polyp.
  – Switch on the cutting and coagulation current.
  – Retrieve the severed polyp.
▶ Inspect the resection site.

Complications

▶ Bleeding
▶ Perforation

■ Endoscopic Mucosectomy

Key Characteristics

▶ Endoscopic mucosectomy is an increasingly common procedure used for the treatment of early carcinomas in the esophagus and stomach.

Indications

▶ Early esophageal carcinomas confined to the mucosa
▶ Small early carcinomas in the stomach
▶ Large adenomas in the stomach

 Technique

▶ Pick up the suspicious mucosa with the biopsy forceps or suck the mucosa into a suction cap.
▶ Place a snare over the raised mucosa and resect the tissue.
▶ Technical details of the procedure are operator-dependent.

■ Photodynamic Therapy

Key Characteristics

▶ A photosensitizing agent is administered that becomes concentrated in the malignant or premalignant lesion.
▶ Several agents are available: dihematoporphyrin ether, 5-aminolevulinic acid (5-ALA), and meta-tetra(hydroxyphenyl)chlorin.
▶ Several hours after the agent is administered, light is applied locally to induce a photochemical reaction leading to tissue necrosis.

Indications

▶ Dysplasia and early carcinoma in the setting of Barrett esophagus
▶ Early esophageal carcinoma

Evaluation

▶ Advantage
  – Suitable for inoperable patients
▶ Disadvantages
  – The lesion is destroyed and therefore unavailable for histological processing and definitive staging.
  – High costs and problems with dose adjustment

Foreign Body Removal

■ Incidence and Location

It is common for foreign bodies to be swallowed, and 70% of the patients are children. Approximately 80–90% of swallowed objects will pass spontaneously through the gastrointestinal tract, while 10–20% will need to be removed endoscopically. One percent will require surgical removal. Swallowed objects most frequently become lodged at the physiological constrictions of the esophagus and at sites of abnormal narrowing (strictures, rings, or malignant tumors).

■ Symptoms

The complaints are highly variable and can range from essentially no complaints, a globus sensation, or retrosternal pain to signs of complete esophageal obstruction or perforation. Objects that pass through the lower esophageal sphincter will usually be eliminated by the natural route.

Injuries from swallowed objects may be caused by pressure necrosis (coins, etc.), pricks and lacerations (needles, razor blades), or toxins (batteries, drug-packed condoms).

■ Rules for Management

Indications

Endoscopic **foreign body removal** is recommended for:
▶ Objects that are sharp or pointed, larger than 2 cm or longer than 5 cm, and for toxic objects
▶ All foreign bodies that are stuck in the esophagus
▶ Patients who have had gastrointestinal surgery
▶ Patients with prior diseases of the gastrointestinal tract

A **wait-and-see approach** is recommended for objects that are round or blunt, smaller than 2 cm or shorter than 5 cm, and nontoxic. The patient should be observed for 10 days. If the foreign body is still detectable within the stomach at that time, it should be retrieved endoscopically.

Prior to Endoscopy

▶ Plain chest radiograph (no contrast medium due to risk of aspiration)
▶ Plain abdominal radiograph
▶ Assess the need for intubation (especially with foreign bodies that are difficult to grasp).
▶ If possible, perform a trial run using a duplicate object.
▶ Check the indication for surgical removal.

Materials

A range of different instruments are available for foreign body retrieval (Fig. 4.**30**):
▶ Foreign-body grasping forceps
▶ Polyp forceps
▶ Stone-retrieval baskets
▶ Esophageal dilating balloons
▶ Snares

Follow-Up

▶ Clinical follow-up visits
▶ Radiographic follow-ups (perforation?)

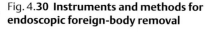

Fig. 4.**30 Instruments and methods for endoscopic foreign-body removal**

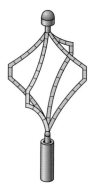 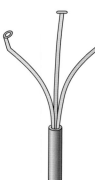 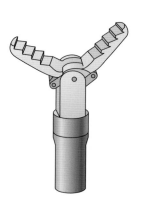 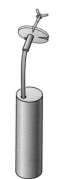 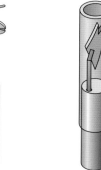 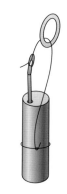

a Stone-retrieval basket for extracting foreign bodies

b Triprong grasper for extracting round foreign bodies

c Toothed forceps for removing small irregular objects

d Method for retrieving the bumper from a cut PEG tube

e An overtube is used when removing sharp or jagged objects

f Method for removing an object with a hole in it

Foreign Body Removal: Types of Objects Swallowed

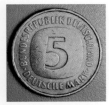

Fig. 4.**31** **Objects that may be swallowed**
a Coins

■ Coins (Fig. 4.31 a)

▶ Remove only if stuck in the esophagus.
▶ Often become trapped at the upper esophageal sphincter.
▶ Coins in the stomach will usually pass spontaneously.

Instruments

▶ Coins with a raised edge: foreign-body grasping forceps
▶ Coins without a raised edge: grasping forceps with a rubber-shod grasping surface

■ Marbles (Fig. 4.31 b)

▶ Try to remove quickly, as they may release toxic substances.

Instruments

▶ Stone-retrieval basket with an overtube
▶ Esophageal dilating balloon (only after intubation)

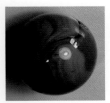

b Marbles

■ Batteries (Fig. 4.31 c, d)

▶ Try to remove quickly, as batteries release heavy metals.
▶ Potassium or sodium hydroxide, burns

Instruments

▶ Stone-retrieval basket with an overtube
▶ Esophageal dilating balloon (only after intubation)

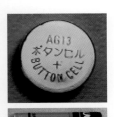

c, d Batteries

■ Pieces of Meat (Fig. 4.31 e)

▶ Common in adults
▶ Many patients have a distal stricture due to reflux esophagitis.

Instruments

▶ Stone-retrieval basket
▶ Suction at the tip of an overtube
▶ **Caution:** Pushing a piece of meat down into the stomach is risky due to the perforation hazard!

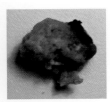

e Piece of meat

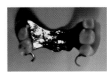

f Partial denture

■ Partial Dentures (Fig. 4.31 f)

▶ Many partial dentures have sharp hooks.

Instruments

▶ Foreign-body grasping forceps
▶ Snare
▶ Stone-retrieval basket
▶ All instruments should be used with an overtube.

■ Needles, Toothpicks
(Fig. 4.**31 g**)

▶ Often difficult to locate

Instruments

▶ Grasping forceps
▶ Snare with overtube
▶ Remove with the point trailing.

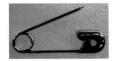

g Safety pin

■ Foreign Bodies with a Hole
(Fig. 4.**31 h**)

▶ Easy to remove

Instruments

▶ Thread and grasping forceps

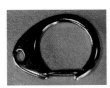

h Metal object with a hole

■ Percutaneous Endoscopic Gastronomy (PEG) Bumper
(Fig. 4.**31 i**)

▶ The internal bumper of the PEG should be removed after cutting the tube.

Instruments

▶ Open biopsy forceps
▶ Snare

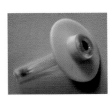

i PEG bumper

■ Condoms Containing Narcotics (Fig. 4.**31 j**)

▶ Endoscopic retrieval is very risky.
▶ Surgical removal is safest for most patients.

Instruments

▶ Removal with a snare may be tried.

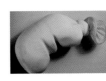

j Drug-filled condom

4

PEG Placement: Principle, Indications, and Contraindications

■ Principle

PEG provides a rapid, simple method for long-term enteral feeding. Although the method can generally be used without complications, there are still some significant risks that should be kept in mind.

> PEG placement is a technically simple procedure (Figs. 4.**32**, 4.**33**). A cannula is passed through the abdominal wall, and a guide suture is threaded into the stomach through the cannula. It is retrieved endoscopically, withdrawn through the mouth, and used to pull the PEG tube down the esophagus and through the anterior abdominal wall, where it is anchored in place.

PEG placement can usually be performed under conscious sedation, but selected cases may require general anesthesia. If the patient has had a gastrectomy, the tube may also be placed in a loop of jejunum (percutaneous endoscopic jejunostomy [PEJ]), in the duodenum, or in an interposed colon segment (Figs. 4.**35**–4.**37**).

■ PEG Tubes

PEG tubes are available in various sizes and designs.

In the simplest case, the tube ends at the retention bumper on the inner wall of the stomach. If the tube is large enough, a second, thinner tube can be threaded through the gastrostomy tube and placed endoscopically in the duodenum to reduce the risk of aspiration (Fig. 4.**34**). From there the tube will be carried into the jejunum by spontaneous peristalsis. All-in-one tubes with an internal component that is placed endoscopically in the duodenum are not recommended because they may bend back toward the esophagus, creating a risk of aspiration.

■ Alternative Methods of Tube Placement

Computed tomography (CT)–guided gastrostomy and ultrasound-guided gastrostomy are options that may be considered in cases where endoscopy cannot be performed.

■ Indications

A PEG tube is indicated for maintaining enteral nutrition in patients with swallowing difficulties, alimentary obstructions, or wasting diseases. PEG placement in geriatric patients with multiple morbidity is problematic. The indications are reviewed in Table 4.**10**.

■ Contraindications

PEG placement is contraindicated in moribund patients, in certain types of comorbidity, and in cases where the procedure cannot be done for technical reasons (Table 4.**11**).

■ Informed Consent

Written informed consent should be obtained at least 24 hours before the procedure. Disclosure should be in accordance with general rules and should include a reference to other treatment options.

■ Complications

Mild complaints, especially pain and local inflammation at the puncture site, are not uncommon and are seen in up to 10% of patients. The mortality figures range from 0.5% to 2%, depending on the population, but are significant. Serious complications are technical or infectious in nature (Table 4.**12**; Fig. 4.**38**).

■ Preparations

- Check the indications and contraindications.
- Obtain blood count and coagulation status.
- Discontinue proton pump inhibitors (PPI) and H2 blockers 48 hours before PEG placement.
- Obtain written informed consent 24 hours before the procedure.
- Provide antibiotic coverage if desired (e.g., metronidazole and cefotaxim).
- Patient should fast for 12 hours before the procedure.

■ Aftercare

- No solid foods for a variable period (six hours to three days after PEG placement)
- Afterward, use the tube to feed a gradually progressive diet.
- Check the wound daily.
- After two days, reexamine by endoscopy.

Table 4.**10**   **Indications for PEG placement**

- Neurogenic dysphagia
  - Multiple sclerosis
  - Amyotrophic lateral sclerosis
  - Stroke
- Malignant obstruction
  - ENT malignancy
  - Esophageal carcinoma
  - Gastric carcinoma
- Oncological diseases not affecting the alimentary tract
- HIV infection
- Chronic inflammatory bowel disease
- Cystic fibrosis

Table 4.**11**   **Contraindications to PEG placement**

- Very short life expectancy
- Comorbidity
  - Sepsis
  - Coagulation disorders
  - Multisystem failure
  - Bowel obstruction
  - Peritonitis
  - Ascites
  - Peritoneal carcinomatosis
- Stomach inaccessible for percutaneous puncture
- Inability to transilluminate the stomach wall
- Certain types of prior gastric surgery

Table 4.**12**   **Complications of PEG placement**

- Technical complications
  - Aspiration
  - Faulty puncture technique
  - Perforation
  - Bleeding
  - Leak
- Infections
  - Generalized peritonitis
  - Wound infection

PEG Placement: Technique (1)

Fig. 4.**32**

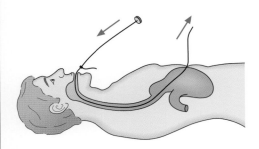

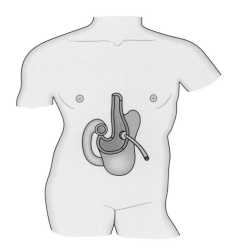

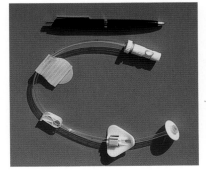

a A heavy-gauge suture is passed through the abdominal wall into the stomach, retrieved endoscopically, and brought out through the mouth. The tube is tied to the suture and pulled down the esophagus into the stomach, where the internal bumper engages against the stomach wall

b The PEG tube in place

c Components of the PEG tube

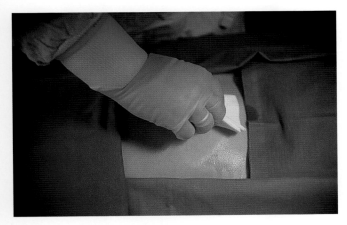

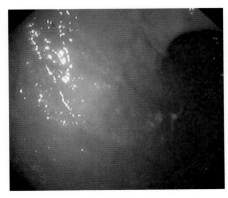

Fig. 4.**33 Technique of PEG placement**
a The puncture site is aseptically prepared and draped. The examination room is darkened

b The endoscope is advanced into the stomach

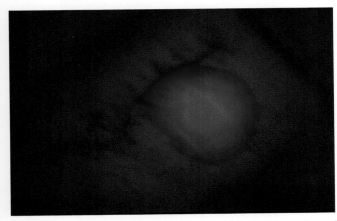

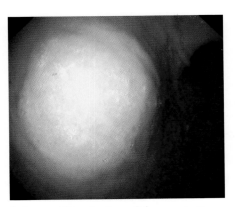

c The puncture site is illuminated from within the stomach, and the abdominal wall is observed for transillumination

d Internal illumination of the puncture site is maintained

PEG Placement: Technique (2)

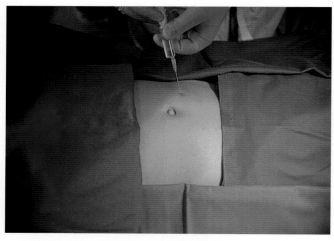

e The skin is infiltrated with local anesthetic. The anesthesia needle is carefully advanced with injection/aspiration until air is aspirated

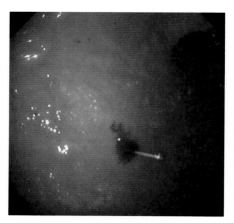

f The tip of the anesthesia needle is identified

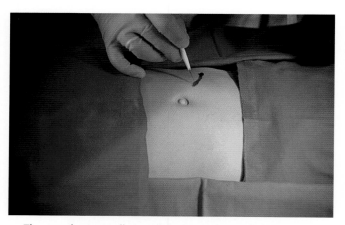

g The anesthesia needle is withdrawn, and a small skin incision is made

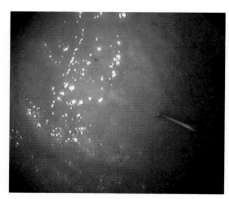

h The proposed puncture site is observed

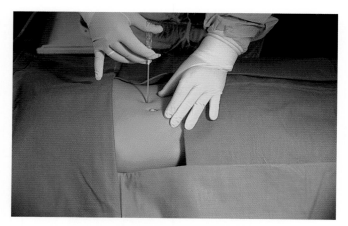

i THe puncture needle is carefully pushed through the abdominal wall (hollow metal stylet with outer plastic cannula)

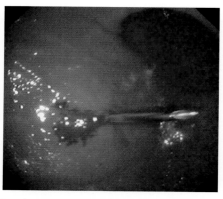

j The puncture needle is identified

PEG Placement: Technique (3)

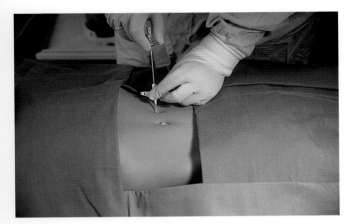

k The stylet is withdrawn while the plastic cannula is carefully advanced

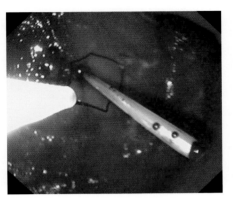

l The plastic cannula is visualized, and a snare is looped around it

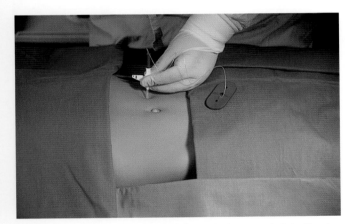

m The passing suture is threaded through the cannula into the stomach

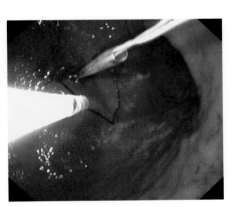

n The passing suture is snared

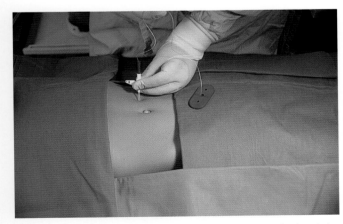

o The assistant carefully feeds the suture from outside the abdomen

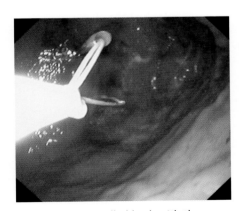

p The suture is pulled back with the endoscope

PEG Placement: Technique (4)

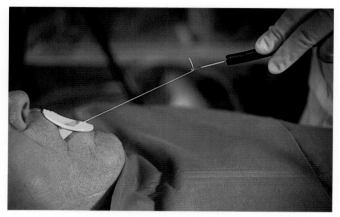

q The endoscope and snared suture are withdrawn through the mouth

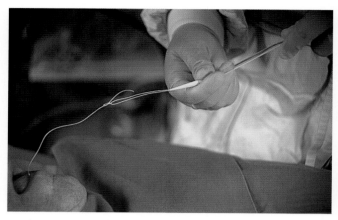

r The suture is tied to the PEG tube

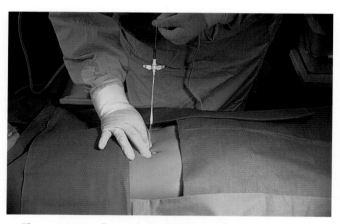

s The assistant pulls gently but briskly on the other end of the suture

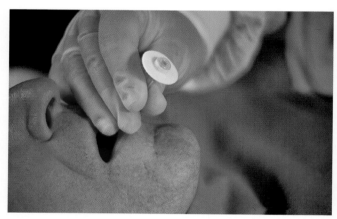

t The PEG tube is stabilized as it enters the mouth

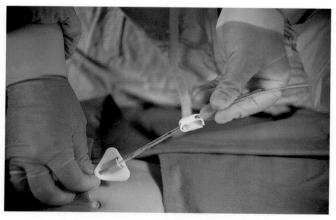

u After the tube has been pulled into place, an external bolster is applied

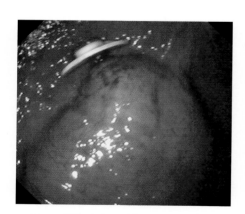

v View of the internal bumper on the stomach wall

Duodenal Tube: Insertion through a PEG

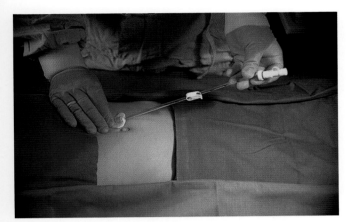

w The tube is tightened to eliminate slack

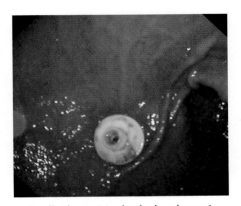

x Finally the PEG is checked endoscopically for correct placement

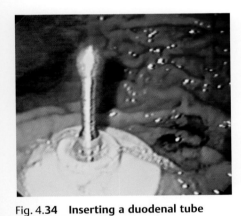

Fig. 4.34 Inserting a duodenal tube through a PEG tube already in place

a The endoscope is advanced to the PEG tube, and the duodenal tube is introduced

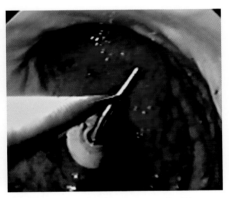

b The duodenal tube is grasped with a forceps

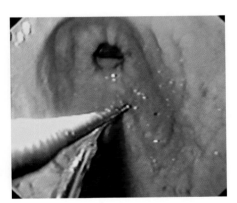

c The endoscope is advanced distally with the grasped duodenal tube

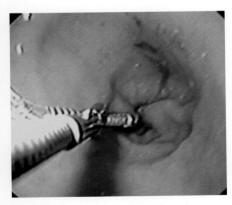

d The endoscope is advanced to the pylorus

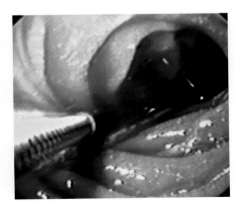

e The endoscope is passed deep into the duodenum, carrying the duodenal tube with it

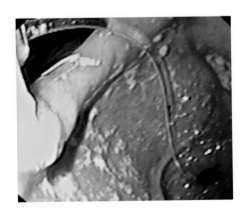

f View of the tube positioned in the duodenum

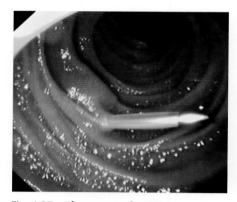

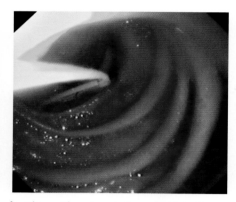

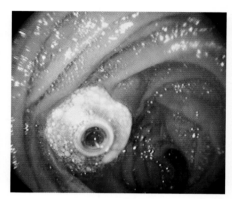

Fig. 4.35 Placement of a PEJ
a The puncture needle is passed into a loop of jejunum

b The guide suture is threaded into the jejunum and grasped

c View of the bumper on the wall of the jejunum

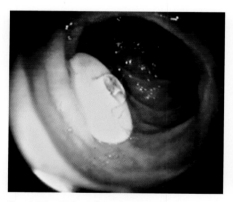

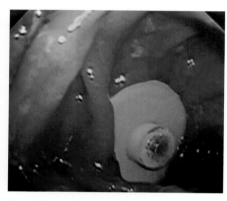

Fig. 4.36 Tube placed in an interposed colon segment

Fig. 4.37 Tube placed in the duodenum of a patient with a Billroth I gastroduodenostomy

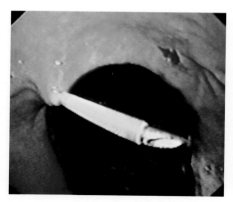

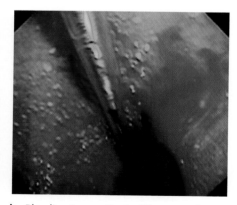

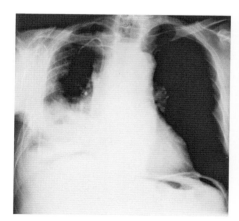

Fig. 4.38 Complications of PEG placement
a Injury to the opposite stomach wall due to insufficient air insufflation

b Bleeding in a patient with a coagulation defect

c Perforation, with free air below the diaphragm

Removal of PEG Tube, Placement of Duodenal Tube

▪ PEG Tube Removal

> A PEG tube can easily be removed when no longer needed (Fig. 4.**39**). It is recommended that the internal bumper be removed endoscopically. After the gastroscope is inserted, the tube is loosened and the bumper is snared. Next, the external portion of the tube is cut and the tube is retrieved endoscopically. Once the tube has been cut, it can easily be retrieved with a snare or with a biopsy forceps, which is passed into the hole of the bumper and then opened. Bumpers that are not retrieved endoscopically are usually passed spontaneously.

Tubes that have been in place for less than 10 days should not be removed due to the risk of peritonitis. Solid foods should be withheld for at least 24 hours after tube removal. An overgrown bumper cannot be removed endoscopically (Fig. 4.**40**).

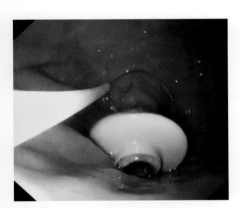 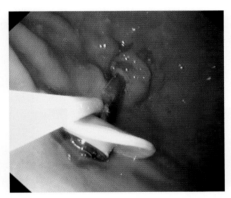 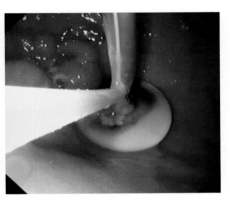

Fig. 4.39 Endoscopic removal of a PEG tube
a The tube is carefully advanced into the stomach from the outside and encircled with a snare

b The snare is tightened on the tube

c The tube is cut from the outside and retrieved with the endoscope

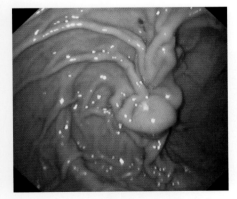

Fig. 4.40 Overgrown bumper. The tube cannot be removed endoscopically

▪ Placement of a Duodenal Tube

Feeding tubes can be placed endoscopically within the duodenum (Fig. 4.**41**). Duodenal tube placement may be necessary in intensive care patients and in ventilated patients with gastric atony that would preclude correct tube placement by a different route.

> The procedure is technically simple. First the endoscope is advanced into the duodenum. Next a guide wire is passed down the working channel and placed deep in the duodenum. The endoscope is then withdrawn while the wire is simultaneously advanced to maintain its position in the duodenum. The endoscope is removed, leaving the proximal end of the wire protruding from the mouth. The wire is rerouted through the nose before attaching it to a feeding tube.

Duodenal Tube Placement: Technique (1)

The nonendoscopic photos on duodenal tube placement in Figure 4.**41** are presented with the kind permission of Mr. Horst Wesche DGPh et al. of Hanover.

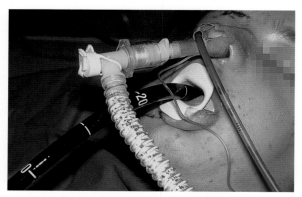

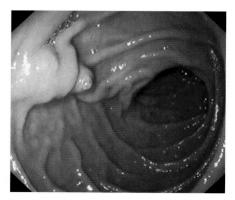

Fig. 4.41   Placement of a duodenal feeding tube

a   The patient is intubated and ventilated. A gastric drainage tube is also visible. The bite guard is inserted, and the endoscope is passed

b   The endoscope is advanced deep into the duodenum

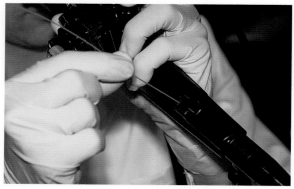

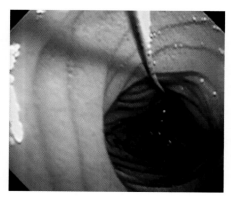

c   A guide wire is passed down the working channel of the endoscope

d   View of the guide wire in the duodenum

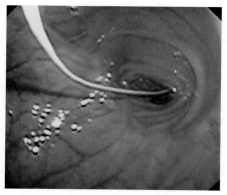

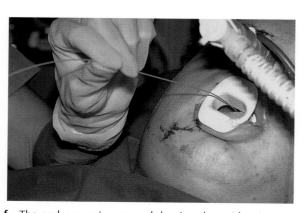

e   While the endoscope is withdrawn, the wire is carefully advanced so that it remains in position

f   The endoscope is removed, leaving the guide wire extending from the mouth

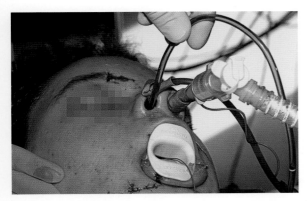

g A tube for rerouting the guide wire is inserted transnasally

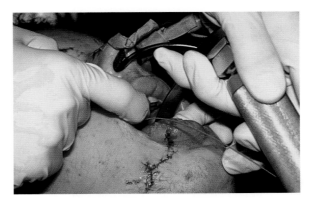

h The pharynx is visualized with a laryngoscope

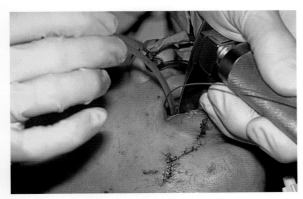

i Secretions are suctioned from the pharynx

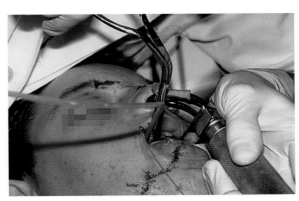

j The rerouting tube is grasped with a Magill forceps and brought out through the mouth

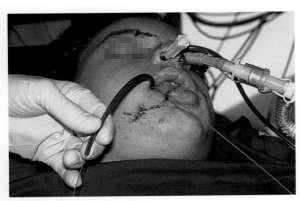

k The ends of the tube now project from the nose and mouth in a U shape. The guide wire is inserted

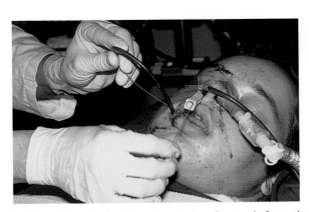

l The guide wire has been inserted and extends from the rerouting tube, which is visible in the right nostril

Duodenal Tube Placement: Technique (3)

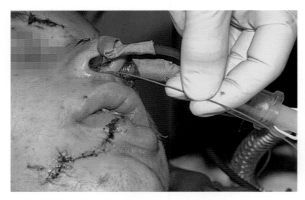

m The reroute is completed by withdrawing the tube and guide wire through the nose

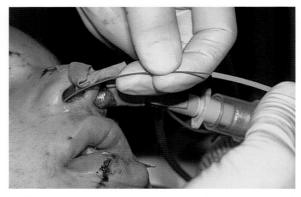

n The feeding tube is advanced over the extracorporeal part of the guide wire. At this time the guide wire must be secured at the nose to prevent dislodgment

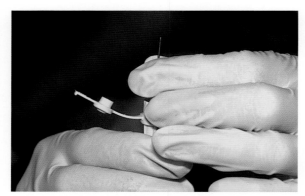

o The feeding tube has been advanced over the guide wire but is still outside the body. The guide wire projects from the end of the tube

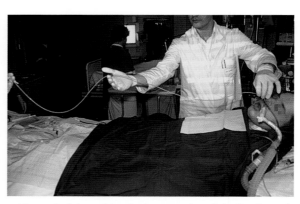

p The end of the guide wire is grasped, and the feeding tube is carefully threaded over the transnasal guide wire into the gastrointestinal tract

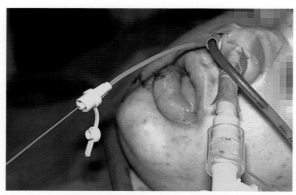

q The feeding tube has been advanced into the duodenum. The guide wire is still inside the tube

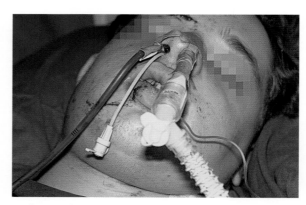

r The wire has been removed, leaving the feeding tube in a functional position within the duodenum. Tube placement should still be checked radiographically, however

Upper Gastrointestinal Stenoses, Malignant Strictures

■ Causes and Sites of Occurrence

Stenoses in the upper gastrointestinal tract can result from benign and malignant diseases. The causes are listed in Table 4.**13**. The most frequent site of occurrence is the esophagus. A less common site is the gastric outlet. Significant stenoses of the duodenum, usually a result of adjacent malignancies, are very rare (Table 4.**14**).

Table 4.**13** **Causes of upper gastrointestinal stenoses**

> ▶ Benign
> - Inflammatory, cicatricial: peptic stricture, corrosive ingestion, radiation
> - Neurogenic: achalasia
> - Postoperative: fundoplication, tight anastomosis after resection
> - Postinterventional: banding of esophageal varices
> ▶ Malignant
> - Esophageal carcinoma
> - Bronchial carcinoma compressing the esophagus
> - Malignant stricture of the gastric outlet

Table 4.**14** **Location of upper gastrointestinal stenoses**

> ▶ Esophagus
> ▶ Gastroesophageal junction
> ▶ Pylorus

Table 4.**15** **Treatment of upper gastrointestinal stenoses**

> ▶ Expansion techniques
> - Bougie dilation
> - Balloon dilation
> - Incision
> ▶ Implantation techniques
> - Tube implantation
> - Implantation of self-expanding stents
> ▶ Tumor ablation
> - Laser
> - Argon plasma coagulation
> ▶ Pharmacological
> - Botulinum toxin
> ▶ Feeding tubes
> - PEG

■ Treatment Options

Treatment options for upper gastrointestinal stenoses include surgical techniques, endoscopic techniques to restore patency, and feeding tube placement (PEG, see p. 160). The treatment of choice depends on the benign or malignant nature of the stenosis, its location, the operability of the patient, and the technical capabilities of the department. The endoscopic treatment options for upper gastrointestinal stenoses are reviewed in Table 4.**15**.

■ Malignant Strictures

Esophageal and bronchial carcinoma are the most frequent causes of malignant strictures in the upper gastrointestinal tract.

■ Esophageal Carcinoma (Figs. 4.**42**, 4.**43**)

Less than 50 % of squamous cell carcinomas of the esophagus are operable when diagnosed. The five-year survival rate is very poor, at less than 20 %. One should be cautious in selecting these patients for palliative procedures.

 Endoscopic treatment options

> ▶ Stent implantation (treatment of choice)
> ▶ Tube implantation
> ▶ Laser therapy (especially for short strictures)
> ▶ Bougie dilation (as a prelude to stenting, intubation, or laser therapy)

■ Bronchial Carcinoma (Fig. 4.**44**)

Advanced bronchial carcinoma can lead to severe compression and infiltration of the esophagus with luminal obstruction.

 Endoscopic treatment options

> ▶ Stent implantation
> ▶ Tube implantation
> ▶ **Caution:** Laser treatment is contraindicated due to the risk of fistula formation.

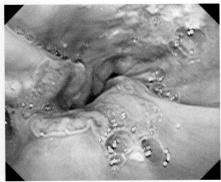

Fig. 4.**42** **Esophageal stricture caused by squamous cell carcinoma**

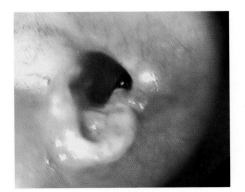

Fig. 4.**43** **Squamous cell carcinoma.** Recurrent tumor

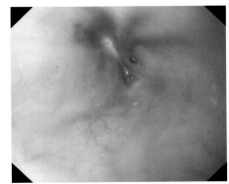

Fig. 4.**44** **Bronchial carcinoma.** The tumor has infiltrated and compressed the esophagus

Benign Stenoses

■ Peptic Esophageal Stricture (Fig. 4.45)

Peptic strictures of the esophagus are a complication of untreated reflux esophagitis.

 Endoscopic treatment options
▶ Bougie dilation
▶ Balloon dilation

■ Gastric Outlet Stricture

Gastric outlet stricture is usually a complication of recurrent gastric ulcers.

 Endoscopic treatment options
▶ Balloon dilation

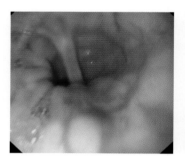

Fig. 4.**45** **Peptic stricture**

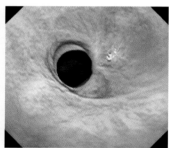

Fig. 4.**46** **Stricture due to caustic ingestion**

■ Corrosive Ingestion (Fig. 4.**46**)

Strictures can develop as a late complication of corrosive ingestion, causing luminal obstruction.

 Endoscopic treatment options
▶ Bougie dilation
▶ Balloon dilation

■ Radiation

Radiation injury of the esophagus following radiotherapy to the lung or mediastinum can lead to cicatricial strictures.

 Endoscopic treatment options
▶ Bougie dilation

■ Achalasia (Fig. 4.**47**)

Achalasia is a neurogenic disorder characterized by a failure of relaxation of the lower esophageal sphincter.

 Endoscopic treatment options
▶ Balloon dilation (treatment of choice)
▶ Injection of botulinum toxin (experimental)

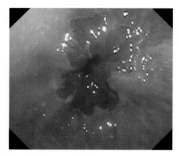

Fig. 4.**47** **Achalasia**

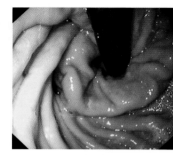

Fig. 4.**48** **Fundoplication**

■ Fundoplication (Fig. 4.**48**)

Postoperative stenosis can occur as a possible complication of fundoplication.

 Endoscopic treatment options
▶ Bougie dilation
▶ Balloon dilation

■ Anastomotic Stenosis (Fig. 4.**49**)

The anastomoses that are performed in upper gastrointestinal resections (gastric resection, cardiectomy) may become stenotic, producing obstructive symptoms.

 Endoscopic treatment options
▶ Bougie dilation
▶ Balloon dilation

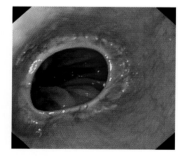

Fig. 4.**49** **Tight anastomosis following esophageal resection**

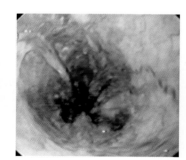

Fig. 4.**50** **Stricture following multiple sclerotherapy injections**

■ Banding and Sclerotherapy of Varices (Fig. 4.**50**)

Cicatricial strictures can develop as a late complication following the banding or sclerotherapy of esophageal varices.

 Endoscopic treatment options
▶ Bougie dilation
▶ Balloon dilation

Upper Gastrointestinal Stenoses: Dilation Methods

■ Bougie Dilation

Principle and Key Characteristics

▶ Principle: Tapered bougies in graduated sizes are passed over a guide wire, converting longitudinal forces into radial forces that dilate the stricture.
▶ Disadvantages
  – Laborious
  – Requires frequent repetition

Indications

▶ Benign cicatricial strictures in the esophagus
  – Peptic strictures
  – Postoperative strictures
▶ Malignant strictures, before implanting a prosthesis

Materials

▶ Savary bougies, 5–20 mm in diameter
▶ Eder–Puestow dilators
▶ Other dilators

▦ Technique

▶ Pass a guide wire under endoscopic vision.
▶ If endoscopy is not possible, place the guide wire under fluoroscopic guidance.
▶ Check the wire position fluoroscopically.
▶ Carefully insert the smallest bougie.
▶ Check endoscopically for esophageal tears.
▶ Progressively increase the size of the bougies in 1 mm increments.
▶ Pass three dilators per session.
▶ Dilate to a maximum of 12–14 mm

Complications

▶ Perforation
▶ Bleeding

■ Balloon Dilation

Principle and Key Characteristics

▶ Principle: A balloon is passed into the stenosis and inflated.
▶ The inflation exerts radial forces that dilate the stenosis.

Indications

▶ Achalasia (Fig. 4.**51**)
▶ Benign pyloric strictures not treatable with bougies
▶ Benign peptic strictures of the pyloric region
▶ Some malignant strictures

Materials

▶ Balloon catheters of various designs (Fig. 4.**52**)

▦ Technique

▶ Three techniques are available for balloon placement:
  1. Pass a guide wire under endoscopic vision. Remove the endoscope, advance the dilating balloon over the guide wire into the stenosis (through-the-channel, TTC), and inflate the balloon.
  2. Visualize the stenosis endoscopically. Pass a dilating balloon down the instrument channel of the scope and advance it into the stenosis (through-the-scope, TTS). Inflate the balloon.
  3. Mount the dilating balloon on the endoscope, advance the endoscope–balloon assembly into the stenosis, and inflate the balloon.
▶ Pressure: 250–300 mmHg
▶ Duration: one to three minutes

Complications

▶ Perforation
▶ Bleeding

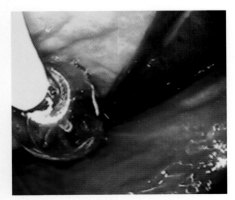

Fig. 4.**51** **Balloon dilation in achalasia.** The endoscope is visible next to the dilating balloon

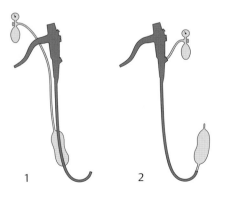
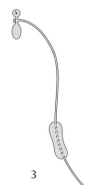

Fig. 4.**52** **Systems for balloon dilation**

Upper Gastrointestinal Stenoses: Incision, Self-Expanding Stents

■ Incision of Strictures

Principle

▶ Incision of the scarred area under endoscopic vision

Indications

▶ Short, annular cicatricial strictures

Materials

▶ Diathermy needle or argon plasma coagulator

Technique

▶ Three or more incisions are made in a stellate pattern under endoscopic vision.

Complications

▶ Perforation
▶ Bleeding

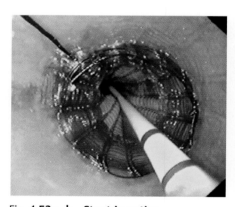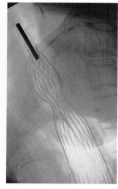

Fig. 4.53 a, b   Stent insertion   b

■ Self-Expanding Stents

Principle

▶ A small-lumen metal mesh stent is introduced, positioned, and released, expanding to a larger luminal size.

Indications

▶ Malignant strictures of the esophagus
▶ Treatment of choice for strictures due to inoperable esophageal carcinoma

Materials

▶ Stent system. Several types are available, including:
  – Strecker stents
  – Wall stents
  – Coated stents
  – Uncoated stents

 Technique (Figs. 4.53–4.56)

▶ Dilate the stricture to 9–10 mm with bougies.
▶ Place a guide wire through the endoscope, aided if necessary by fluoroscopic monitoring.
▶ Locate the upper and lower tumor margins endoscopically or radiographically.
▶ Remove the endoscope.
▶ Introduce the stent system (stent and applicator) over the guide wire.
▶ Release the stent (variable mechanism, depending on the design).

Complications (Figs. 4.57, 4.58)

▶ Chest pain
▶ Failure of stent expansion
▶ Tumor growth into the stent
▶ Overgrowth of the ends of the stent
▶ Dislodgment
▶ Compression by tumor growth

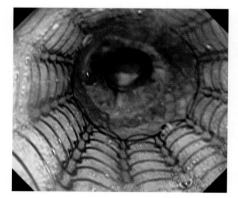

Fig. 4.54   Ultraflex stent

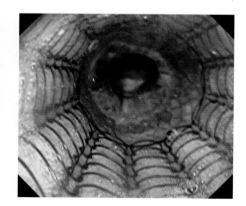

Fig. 4.55   Upper edge of stent

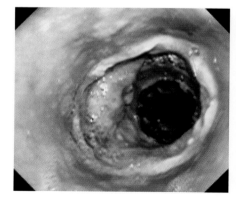

Fig. 4.56   Overgrown stent

Upper Gastrointestinal Stenoses: Intubation, Laser Treatment

■ Intubation

Principle and Key Characteristics

▶ Principle: insertion of a molded plastic tube into a stricture
▶ Established, economical treatment method
▶ Increasingly superseded by self-expanding stents
▶ Disadvantages
  – Frequently requires general anesthesia.
  – Stricture must be dilated to 15–18 mm before intubation.

Indications

▶ Malignant esophageal strictures with or without a fistula
▶ Long, circumferential strictures without angulation
▶ Malignant strictures of the gastric cardia

Materials

▶ Plastic tube (many different types are available)
▶ Graduated bougies
▶ Guide wire
▶ Pusher

 Technique

▶ Dilate the stricture to 15–18 mm with graduated bougies.
▶ Locate the proximal and distal tumor margins endoscopically.
▶ Pass the guide wire down the endoscope.
▶ Remove the endoscope, leaving the guide wire in place.
▶ Assemble the delivery system (e.g., bougie, tube, and pusher).
▶ Introduce the delivery system with the tube.
▶ Advance through the stricture.
▶ Remove the bougie, pusher, and guide wire.

Complications

▶ Perforation
▶ Bleeding
▶ Dislodgment
▶ Tube obstruction

■ Laser Treatment

Principle and Key Characteristics

▶ Principle: tumor tissue is coagulated with a Nd:YAG laser to restore patency.
▶ Disadvantage
  – Relatively long duration of treatment (up to four weeks)

Indications

▶ Stricture caused by exophytic tumor growth
▶ Short strictures in particular

Contraindications

▶ Fistula
▶ Luminal narrowing due to extrinsic compression

Materials

▶ Nd:YAG laser

 Technique

▶ Advance the endoscope to the stricture.
▶ Introduce the laser probe, advance it to the stricture.
▶ Laser the tumor tissue in short bursts.
▶ Repeat at intervals of several days.

4

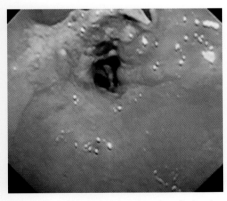

Fig. 4.**57** **Compression of an implanted stent by tumor growth**

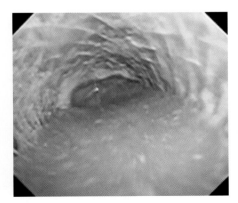

Fig. 4.**58** **Gastroesophageal reflux following stent insertion**

Upper Gastrointestinal Stenoses: Coagulation and Botulinum Toxin

■ Argon Plasma Coagulation

Principle and Key Characteristics

▶ Principle: high-frequency energy is transmitted to the lesion through argon gas, coagulating the tissue without direct contact.
▶ The effect is relatively superficial, so there is less risk of perforation than with a laser.

Indications

▶ Malignant strictures

 Technique

▶ Advance the endoscope to the stricture.
▶ Insert the probe to within a few millimeters of the stricture.
▶ Coagulate the tumor tissue, then stop due to the low penetration depth.
▶ Repeat the treatment at intervals of several days.

■ Injection of Botulinum Toxin

Principle and Key Characteristics

▶ Principle: botulinum toxin very selectively inhibits acetylcholine release at cholinergic nerve endings, diminishing excitatory nerve impulses in the gastrointestinal tract.
▶ Injection into the lower esophageal sphincter induces temporary, reversible relaxation of the sphincter muscles.
▶ Disadvantage
  – Effect lasts for approximately two to six months, rarely for 12 months.

Indications

▶ Achalasia (experimental)

Contraindications

▶ Myasthenia gravis
▶ Motor neuron disorders
▶ Pregnancy and nursing
▶ Concurrent use of other medications (aminoglycosides, calcium antagonists)

Materials

▶ Botulinum toxin

 Technique

▶ Advance the endoscope to the lower esophageal sphincter.
▶ Inject a total of 100 I.U. of botulinum toxin into the four quadrants of the esophageal sphincter.

Complications

▶ Reflux following treatment

Chromoendoscopy: Lugol Solution

Most gastrointestinal tumors are diagnosed at a fairly advanced stage and consequently have a poor prognosis. Since early carcinomas have a very favorable prognosis, early diagnosis is of key importance in reducing the mortality from gastrointestinal tumors. It has been shown that the early diagnosis of epithelial gastrointestinal tumors can be improved by the use of chromoendoscopy and magnification endoscopy.

■ Definition and Stains

Chromoendoscopy refers to the intravital staining of epithelial structures during the endoscopic examination. Several types of stain are used in chromoendoscopy: absorptive, contrast, and reactive (Table 4.**16**). Absorptive stains are taken up by special epithelial cells and can differentiate cells according to whether they are stained or unstained. Contrast stains cause relatively marked enhancement of intestinal mucosa and are often used in magnification endoscopy. Reactive stains are used to identify certain secretions in which the stain induces a color reaction.

At present, the chromoendoscopy of Barrett esophagus is of greatest importance in the upper gastrointestinal tract (Table 4.**17**).

Table 4.**16** **Stains used in chromoendoscopy**

> ▶ Absorptive stains
>   – Lugol solution
>   – Methylene blue
>   – Toluidine blue
> ▶ Contrast stains
>   – Indigo carmine
> ▶ Reactive stains
>   – Congo red
>   – Phenol red

Table 4.**17** **Early carcinomas that are accessible to chromoendoscopy**

> ▶ Esophagus
>   – Squamous cell carcinoma
>   – Adenocarcinoma in the distal esophagus (Barrett carcinoma)
> ▶ Stomach
>   – Early carcinoma in high-risk groups (pernicious anemia, operated stomach)

■ Lugol Solution

Principle and Key Characteristics

▶ Principle: Lugol solution is a solution of iodine and potassium iodide. It reacts with the glycogen in the normal squamous epithelium of the esophagus to produce a dark brownish–green stain.
▶ Lugol solution stains healthy squamous epithelial cells in the esophagus.
▶ It does not stain inflammatory, dysplastic, or carcinomatous areas.
▶ Thus, staining with Lugol solution (Fig. 4.**59**) is useful for identifying:
  – Intact squamous epithelium (stained)
  – Abnormal areas within healthy squamous epithelium (unstained)
▶ Inflammatory, dysplastic, and carcinomatous changes cannot be differentiated by their staining properties alone.

 Technique

▶ Irrigate the esophageal mucosa with water.
▶ Apply 1% Lugol solution.
▶ Wait for four minutes.
▶ Inspect the area endoscopically and take selective biopsies.

Indications

▶ Patients at high risk for developing squamous cell carcinoma of the esophagus (preexisting squamous cell carcinoma of the head or neck, achalasia)

Contraindications

▶ Iodine allergy
▶ Hyperthyroidism

Side Effects

▶ Allergy
▶ Pharyngeal irritation

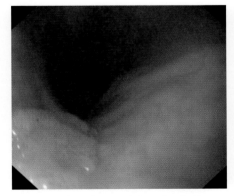
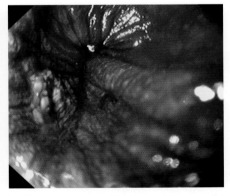

Fig. 4.**59** **Staining with Lugol solution**
a Adenomas in the esophagus

b The squamous epithelium of the esophagus is deeply stained by Lugol solution, while the adenoma is weakly stained

Chromoendoscopy: Methylene Blue

■ Methylene Blue and Barrett Epithelium

Principle and Key Characteristics

▶ Principle: blue-staining absorptive stain
▶ Methylene blue stains:
  – Actively absorbing epithelial cells in the small intestine and colon
  – Areas of complete and incomplete intestinal metaplasia in the esophagus and stomach
▶ It does not stain:
  – Columnar epithelial metaplasia of the fundus and cardia type
  – Squamous epithelium
▶ Tissues showing weak, nonhomogeneous, or no uptake of methylene blue:
  – Dysplasias and carcinomas within actively absorbing epithelium
▶ Barrett epithelium
  – Usually shows a mosaic of columnar epithelial metaplasia of the fundus and cardia type and of the intestinal type. Barrett carcinoma arises predominantly from columnar epithelial metaplasia of the intestinal type.
▶ Thus, methylene blue staining (Figs. 4.**60**, 4.**61**) permits the identification of:
  – Specialized intestinal-type columnar epithelium (positive stain)
  – Dysplasias and early carcinomas for selective biopsy (weak, nonhomogeneous, or no uptake in areas of columnar epithelial metaplasia)

 Technique

▶ Apply acetylcysteine solution to remove superficial mucus.
▶ Wait for two minutes.
▶ Spray with 0.5 % methylene blue solution.
▶ Wait for three minutes.
▶ Rinse with saline solution or water.
▶ Inspect the area endoscopically and take selective biopsies.

Indications

▶ Barrett esophagus

Side Effects

▶ The only side effect is greenish discoloration of the urine.

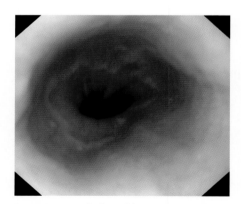

Fig. 4.60 Methylene blue staining of a short Barrett esophagus
a Short Barrett esophagus, unstained

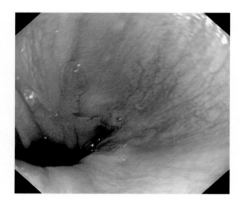

b Magnified view after methylene blue application shows deep blue staining at the right edge of the tonguelike epithelial extension

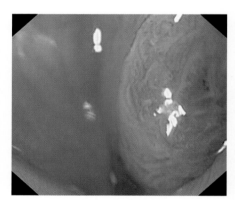

c At higher magnification, the intensely blue-stained area at the right edge of the epithelial extension represents a site of complete intestinal metaplasia

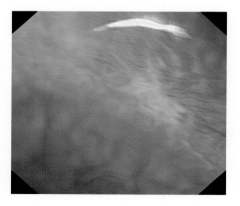

Fig. 4.**61** **Barrett esophagus.** The reddish area on the left represents columnar epithelial metaplasia of the fundus and cardia type. The blue-stained area on the right is intestinal metaplasia. Between them is a pale blue area of dysplasia

Chromoendoscopy: Indigo Carmine, Uses of Vital Stains

■ Indigo Carmine

Principle

▶ Indigo carmine is not absorbed. It is a bluish dye that fills interstices and folds in the mucosa, highlighting surface irregularities and lesions and making them easier to distinguish from their surroundings (Fig. 4.**62**).

 Technique

▶ Irrigate the area with water to remove mucus.
▶ Spray with a 0.1–1 % solution of indigo carmine.
▶ Inspect the area endoscopically and take selective biopsies.

Indications

▶ Identification of early gastric carcinoma
▶ Detection of villous atrophy in the duodenum in celiac disease
▶ Identification and delineation of mucosal lesions in the esophagus

■ Possible Uses of Vital Stains in the Upper Gastrointestinal Tract

Esophagus

▶ **Squamous cell carcinoma.** Possible indications are:
– Screening high-risk patients (e.g., with preexisting squamous cell carcinoma of the head or neck, achalasia, or corrosive ingestion)
– Accurately defining the extent of known early carcinoma prior to endoscopic mucosectomy
▶ Method of choice: Lugol solution
▶ **Adenocarcinoma.** Possible indications are:
– Suspected Barrett epithelium in reflux disease
– Surveillance of known Barrett epithelium to identify premalignant, dysplastic, or early malignant areas
▶ Method of choice: methylene blue staining

Stomach

▶ **Adenocarcinoma.** Possible indications are:
– Screening patients with a high cancer risk (e.g., pernicious anemia, previous partial gastrectomy, etc.)
▶ Method of choice: indigo carmine

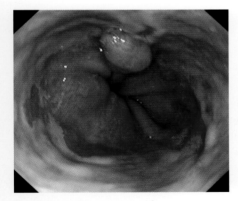 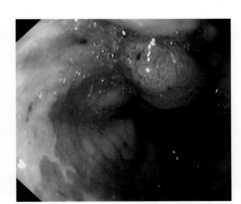 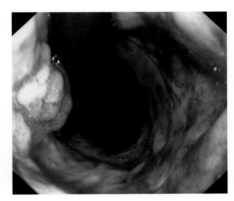

Fig. 4.62 **Indigo carmine dye**
a Polypoid lesions in the distal esophagus, before indigo carmine

b Spraying the area with indigo carmine heightens the contrast between the lesions and their surroundings

c Retroflexed view shows good distal delineation with indigo carmine

Fluorescent Endoscopy and Magnification Endoscopy

Interventional Procedures

■ Principle of Fluorescent Endoscopy

Fluorescent endoscopy is based on the principle that when certain chemical compounds are irradiated with ultraviolet or short-wave light, they emit light at longer wavelengths.

Exogenous fluorescence and autofluorescence. The diagnostic principle of fluorescent endoscopy is based on the differences in fluorescence between normal and abnormal tissues (inflammation, dysplasia, neoplasia, ischemia). In autofluorescence, endogenous substances within the tissue are made to fluoresce, whereas exogenous fluorescence is induced by substances that are added to the tissue, such as 5-ALA. The fluorescence may be demonstrated by spectral analysis or as a fluorescent image.

■ Fluorescent Endoscopy with 5-ALA

 Technique

In fluorescent endoscopy, the tissue is sprayed with 5-ALA, a precursor of the endogenous photosensitizer protoporphyrin IX. It is selectively concentrated in the mucosa, showing a particular affinity for dysplastic or neoplastic areas. The mucosa is probed with a laser fiber, and the fluorescence spectrum is analyzed for an increased concentration of protoporphyrin IX. In a second step, biopsies are taken from any suspicious areas that are identified (Fig. 4.**63**).

Importance

The importance of fluorescent endoscopy in the diagnosis of early neoplastic changes in the esophagus and stomach is currently being evaluated.

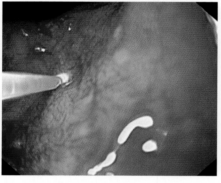
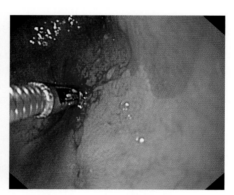

Fig. 4.**63** **Fluorescent endoscopy with 5-ALA**
a The Barrett mucosa is probed after spraying with 5-ALA

b Suspicious areas are identified and biopsied

■ Magnification Endoscopy

Principle. Magnification endoscopy, known also as zoom endoscopy, can be used for the detailed endoscopic evaluation of suspicious areas, especially after staining (Fig. 4.**64**).

Limitations and importance. The main limitation of magnification endoscopy is that the lesions must first be detected by conventional endoscopy before they can be examined under magnification. This problem may be solved by the use of high-resolution instruments (high-resolution endoscopy). The importance of the method in the early detection of malignant lesions is currently being investigated.

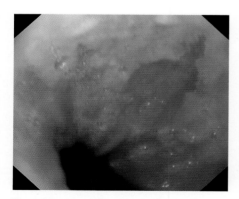
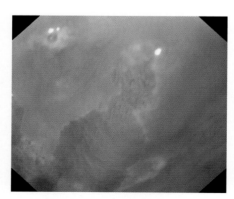
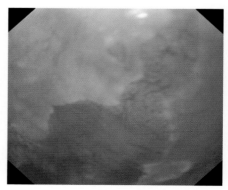

Fig. 4.**64** **Magnification endoscopy**
a Unmagnified view of Barrett epithelium. The area was sprayed with acetic acid to heighten contrast

b Magnified view of the Barrett epithelium

c At higher magnification, the gyriform structure of the Barrett epithelium can be appreciated. Lesions appear as structural irregularities

Enteroscopy

The location of the small intestine makes it difficult to evaluate, especially by diagnostic imaging. The detection of circumscribed pathological changes in the small intestine relies on sonographic, radiographic, scintigraphic, and increasingly on endoscopic techniques (Table 4.**18**).

Table 4.**18** **Techniques for endoscopy of the small intestine**

> ▶ Sonde enteroscopy
> ▶ Push enteroscopy
> ▶ Intraoperative endoscopy
> ▶ Capsule endoscopy

■ Sonde Enteroscopy

▶ Principle: A nondeflectable endoscope is introduced and is carried by peristalsis into the small intestine.
▶ Advantage
 – Relatively deep penetration
▶ Disadvantages
 – Not steerable
 – Limited field of view
 – No interventional options
 – Lengthy procedure (several hours)
 – Uncomfortable procedure

■ Push Enteroscopy

▶ Principle: A steerable endoscope is advanced into the small intestine.
▶ Advantages
 – Relatively well tolerated
 – Relatively short examination time (about 45 minutes)
 – Steerable scope
 – Allows interventional procedures
▶ Disadvantage
 – Limited range (70 cm past the pylorus)

■ Intraoperative Enteroscopy

▶ Principle: The small intestine is surgically exposed, the wall is incised, and the endoscope is manually inserted.
▶ Advantages
 – Only method that ensures complete endoscopic visualization of the small bowel
 – Allows interventional procedures
▶ Disadvantages
 – High cost
▶ Complications
 – Anesthesia risks
 – Surgical risks
 – Endoscopic risks

■ Capsule Endoscopy

▶ Principle: The patient swallows a wireless capsule containing a video imager, light source, and transmitter. The image data are transmitted to a receiver worn on the body.
▶ Advantages
 – Well tolerated
 – Potential visualization of the entire small intestine
▶ Disadvantages
 – Costly
 – Not yet adequately evaluated
 – Does not allow specimen collection

4

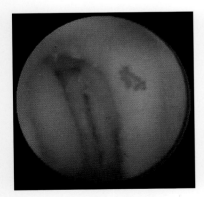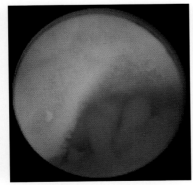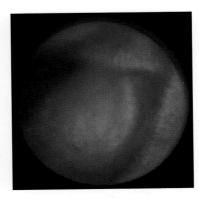

Fig. 4.**65** **Capsule endoscopy**
a Angiodysplasia in the small intestine

b Small oozing hemorrhage in the small intestine

c Polyp in the small intestine

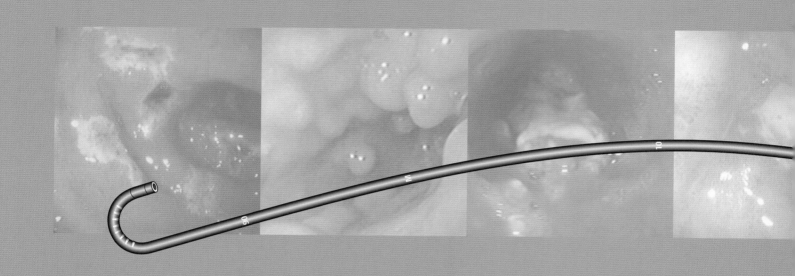

Appendix
Subject Index

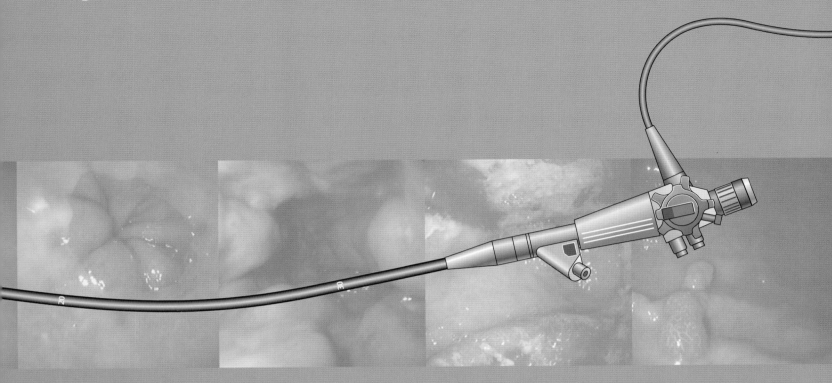

Systematic Endoscopic Examination

An endoscopic examination should be conducted according to a systematic routine. At each point during the examination, the endoscopist should clearly understand what he or she is doing and what he or she is seeing. The sequence of the individual steps will vary somewhat from one examiner to the next, but it is essential to adopt a systematic routine.

The outline below is intended as a practical guide for conducting a systematic endoscopic examination.

Esophagus

1. Upper esophageal sphincter
2. Midesophageal constriction
   - Right main bronchus
   - Aorta
   - Spinal column
3. Retrocardial esophagus
4. Sphincter function
5. Z-line
   - Shape
   - Location in centimeters from the incisors
6. Diaphragmatic hiatus in centimeters from the incisors

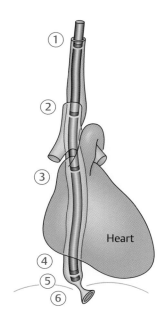

Endoscopic evaluation

▶ Mucosa
   - Color
   - Surface
▶ Shape
   - Symmetry
   - Indentations
▶ Contents
   - Secretions
▶ Peristalsis
   - Frequency
   - Propulsion
   - Symmetry

Stomach

1. Cardia in forward view
2. Body of stomach
   - Greater curvature
   - Lesser curvature
   - Anterior wall
   - Posterior wall
   - Rugal folds
3. Antrum
   - Antral peristalsis
   - Symmetry
4. Pylorus
   - Shape
   - Function
5. Angulus
6. Fundus
7. Cardia in retroflexed view, 360°

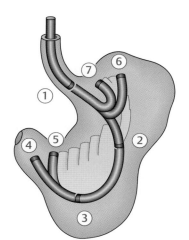

Endoscopic evaluation

▶ Contents
   - Gastric juice
   - Food residues
   - Mucus
▶ Mucosa
   - Color
   - Surface
▶ Identification of adjacent structures
   - Liver
   - Pancreas
   - Spleen
   - Heart
   - Duodenum
▶ Peristalsis

Duodenum

1. Bulb
   - Anterior wall
   - Posterior wall
   - Lesser curvature
   - Greater curvature
2. Descending duodenum
   - Valvulae conniventes
   - Papilla

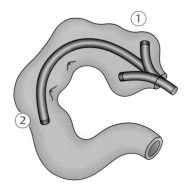

Endoscopic evaluation

▶ Shape
   - Bulb: ulcer niche?
▶ Mucosa
   - Color
   - Surface

Location of Abnormalities

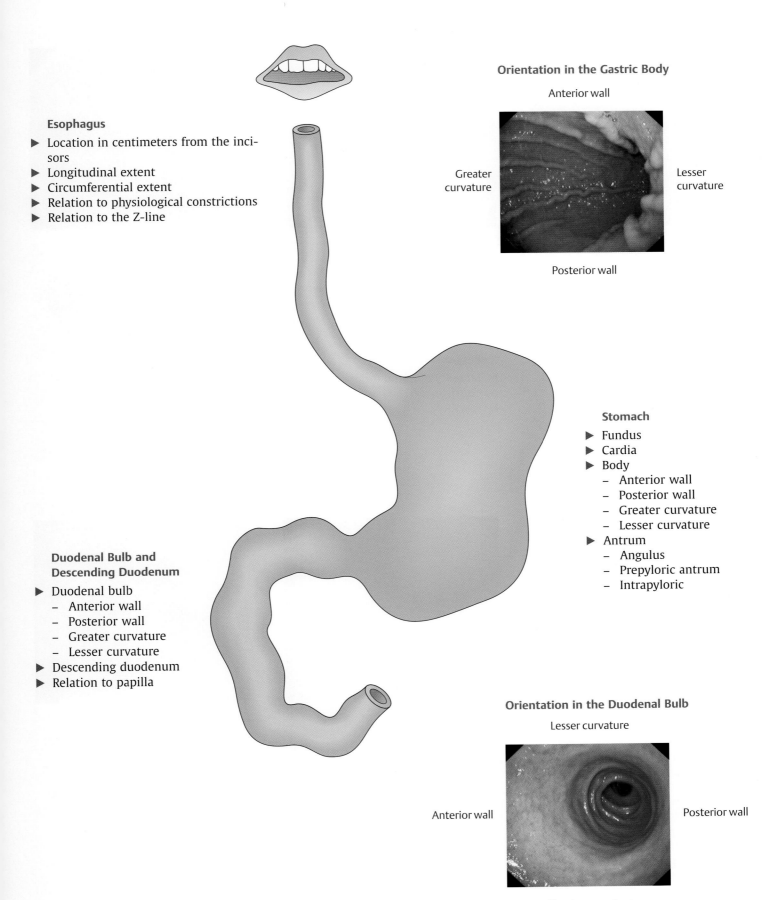

Esophagus
▶ Location in centimeters from the incisors
▶ Longitudinal extent
▶ Circumferential extent
▶ Relation to physiological constrictions
▶ Relation to the Z-line

Orientation in the Gastric Body

Anterior wall

Greater curvature

Lesser curvature

Posterior wall

Stomach
▶ Fundus
▶ Cardia
▶ Body
  – Anterior wall
  – Posterior wall
  – Greater curvature
  – Lesser curvature
▶ Antrum
  – Angulus
  – Prepyloric antrum
  – Intrapyloric

Duodenal Bulb and Descending Duodenum
▶ Duodenal bulb
  – Anterior wall
  – Posterior wall
  – Greater curvature
  – Lesser curvature
▶ Descending duodenum
▶ Relation to papilla

Orientation in the Duodenal Bulb

Lesser curvature

Anterior wall

Posterior wall

Greater curvature

Characterization of Abnormal Findings

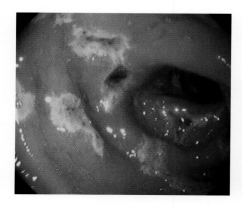
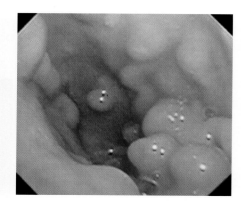
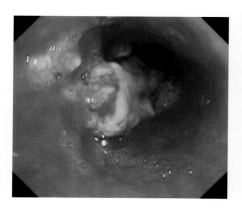

Morphology

- ▶ Size
- ▶ Shape
  - – Oval, round, irregular, spotty, patchy, linear, stippled, confluent
- ▶ Base
  - – Broad, constricted, pedunculated
- ▶ Margins
- ▶ Surface
  - – Smooth, furrowed, glistening, fissured
- ▶ Color
- ▶ Pattern
  - – Coarse, spotty, mottled

Number and Arrangement

- ▶ Number
  - – Solitary, scattered, multiple, numerous, ubiquitous
- ▶ Arrangement
  - – Focal, diffuse

Response to Probing

- ▶ Mobility of lesion or mucosa
- ▶ Consistency
- ▶ Fragility

Stenoses

- ▶ Degree of luminal narrowing
- ▶ Extent
- ▶ Resistance to instrument passage
- ▶ Consistency
- ▶ Mucosal fragility

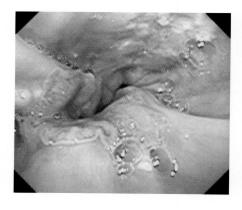
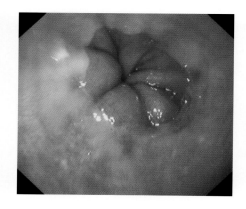
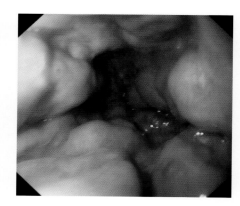

Findings in the Esophagus

- ▶ Carcinoma
  - – Location: in centimeters from the incisors, relation to physiological constrictions, relation to the Z-line
  - – Extent: longitudinal extent, circumferential extent, degree of luminal narrowing
  - – Type of growth
  - – Width of residual lumen
  - – Mobility
  - – Consistency
  - – Fragility

- ▶ Esophagitis
  - – Grade
  - – Extent of lesions
  - – Extent of peptic stricture, if present

- ▶ Varices
  - – Grade
  - – Extent of varices
  - – Signs of increased bleeding risk

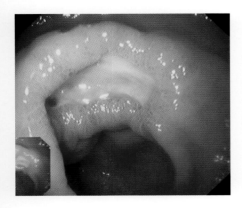 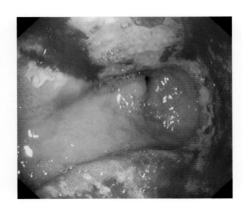 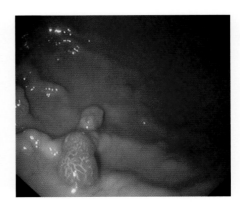

Findings in the Stomach

▶ Erosion, ulcer
  - Location
  - Size
  - Shape: round, oval, linear, bizarre, irregular
  - Number
  - Ulcer base: fibrin, hematin, visible vessel
  - Ulcer margin

▶ Carcinoma
  - Location within the stomach
  - Size
  - Type of growth
  - Consistency
  - Mobility

▶ Polyp
  - Location within the stomach
  - Size
  - Shape
  - Base
  - Surface

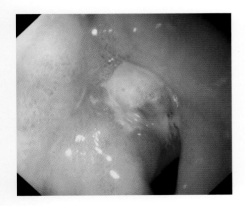 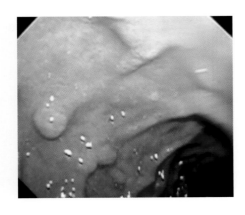

Findings in the Duodenum

▶ Ulcer
  - Location within the bulb
  - Shape: round, oval, linear, bizarre, irregular
  - Number
  - Ulcer base: fibrin, hematin, visible vessel
  - Ulcer margin

▶ Polyp
  - Location within the bulb
  - Size
  - Shape
  - Base
  - Surface

Subject Index

Notes
Page numbers followed by f indicate figures: t indicates tables.
To save space, the following abbreviations have been used:
MALT – mucosa associated lymphoid tissue
PEG – percutaneous endoscopic gastrostomy
vs. indicates a comparison or differential diagnosis